FROM GUT HEALTH TO MENTAL WELLNESS

A FOUR-PART GUIDE THAT USES THE POWER OF THE GUT-BRAIN CONNECTION TO CONQUER STRESS, ANXIETY AND DEPRESSION NATURALLY

HEALTHFIT PUBLISHING

CONTENTS

Free Gut Health Course!

Don't miss out on our exhilarating, FREE course that delves into harnessing gut health for a happier, healthier mind!

Transform Your Life: The Gut-Brain Connection to Mental Wellness

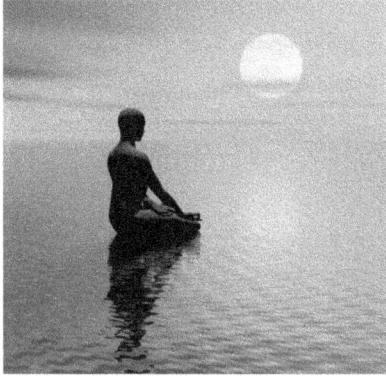

- Unlock the secret to mental wellness with our impactful 10-email course on gut health!
- Learn proven methods to combat stress, anxiety, and depression
- Master mindful eating and stress management
- Build relationships that boost your mental and gut health
- Transform your life with personalized habits for lasting health and happiness

To get your free course, please visit the link or scan the QR code below and let us know the email address to send it to.

pages.healthfitpublishing.com/bonus/fghtmw

Don't miss out!

INTRODUCTION

Your mind and body are intricately linked. This is backed up by science, traditional medicinal theories, and cultural beliefs from around the world. You may even have made the connection through personal physical reactions to mental stimulus.

Have you ever felt butterflies in your stomach when nervous? Have you experienced a 'gut feeling' about a situation, decision, or even another person? These sensations aren't just metaphors, they are hints at a profound truth: our gut and brain are intimately connected. This book delves into this fascinating role of the gut-brain axis. It reveals how our mental state is deeply influenced by our gut health and vice versa.

The idea that the gut and mind interact and influence each other is neither new nor confined to a specific culture or knowledge background. It's a concept that has been iterated across the globe by people from all walks of life. American medical practitioner, Bernie Siegel, wisely noted, 'The mind and body are not separate units, but one integrated system. How we act and what we think, eat, and feel are all related to our health.' Similarly, Sanyasi Satyananda Saraswati, a revered yoga teacher, echoed this sentiment when he expressed, "The mind and body are not separate entities. The gross form of the mind is the body and the subtle form of the body is the mind."

In this guide, we unravel the mysteries of the gut-brain connection. We'll explore how this intricate communication network can be leveraged to nurture and enhance mental and physical wellbeing. By examining the insights science is providing, and using that knowledge to highlight easily actionable strategies, this guide offers a natural holistic approach to managing stress, anxiety, and depression. It's not just about what you eat or how you exercise; it's about understanding the synergy between your mind and gut and harnessing the power of that connection to benefit your wellbeing.

Join us on this enlightening journey to transform your understanding of health and wellness. We're about to bridge the gap between mental and physical health through the power of the gut-brain connection. Let's redefine what it means to be truly healthy from the inside out.

The guide has been created in four parts:

1. Mindfully Supporting Gut Health and Mental Wellness
2. Nutritionally Supporting Gut Health and Mental Wellness
3. Physically Supporting Gut Health and Mental Wellness
4. Mentally and Emotionally Supporting Gut Health and Mental Wellness

Each part focuses on an essential approach to improving overall wellbeing by tapping into and supporting the gut-brain axis. How you work your way through this guide is entirely up to you. There is no single correct approach, but here are some suggestions that might make it easier to adapt it to your personal preferences:

You could read the entire guide through to get a firm grasp of the whole process before deciding how to implement the strategies.

You could follow the guide in sequence, acting on the suggestions as you read through.

If following the parts sequentially isn't for you, why not read the guide through first and then start implementing strategies chronologically or deploy strategies from different parts of the guide in an order that suits you best.

In the last chapter, we discuss how to put all the knowledge you've gained into practice, including how to adjust your gut health and mental wellness journey to suit your own needs.

The key takeaway is that there is no right or wrong way to start making changes to your lifestyle in order to take advantage of the gut-brain axis. The critical factor is making the necessary changes and implementing them in a way that works best for you and supports long-term healthy lifestyle maintenance.

1

THE GUT-MIND CONNECTION

The human body is a genuinely fascinating creation. It's generally accepted that the brain is the boss, controlling numerous bodily functions from breathing to heart rate to emotional responses. As much as the body cannot survive without the brain, this "boss" doesn't independently rule over the body on its own. The brain continually receives messages from tissues, organs, and systems throughout the body. One of these systems is the gastrointestinal tract. Traditional medicine has long recognized the connection between the gut and the brain. Still, from a contemporary scientific medical perspective, it's only recently come into the limelight as a key part of physical and mental health.

THE GUT-BRAIN-AXIS: AN OVERVIEW

The gut-brain axis is the two-way biochemical message highway between the gastrointestinal tract and the central nervous system. It's the signal-relaying mechanism by which the brain and gut send and receive signals from each other. Sometimes, the term is incorrectly applied to gut microbes' vital role in the signaling process. When the gut microbes are expressly included, the term changes to the 'microbiota-gut-brain axis'.

The gut-brain-axis includes the following systems:

- The central nervous system (brain and spinal cord)
- The parasympathetic autonomic nervous system (responsible for involuntary functions when relaxed)
- The sympathetic autonomic nervous system (responsible for involuntary functions in fight-or-flight mode)
- The enteric nervous system (responsible for controlling gut function semi-independently of the brain)
- The vagus nerve (a vital part of the autonomic nervous system)
- The neuroimmune systems (responsible for communication between the immune system and the central nervous system)
- The neuroendocrine system (responsible for the production and release of hormones)
- The hypothalamic–pituitary–adrenal axis

(responsible for regulating physiological stress responses)
- Gut microbiota (the microorganisms inhabiting the gastrointestinal tract)

The Gut Microbiome

A microbiome encompasses all the microorganisms that live within a particular environment as a micro-ecosystem. Microbiota, however, are the microorganisms themselves. A vast number of microbes live in the gastrointestinal tract and are critical for regulating mental and physical health. They are essential players in balancing brain chemistry through the central nervous system. Due to its influence on the brain, the gut is sometimes nicknamed the "second brain," indicating its importance for the brain, and in turn, for mental health.

While there are different species of microbes inhabiting the gut, some of them are incredibly sensitive to changes in the gut microbiome. Disruptions to their environment can significantly impact populations and, therefore, health. Their role in communicating with the brain needs to be explained in order to understand why these microscopic critters are so crucial for maintaining holistic wellbeing.

Communication Between the Gut and Brain

The brain and gut communicate through components of the microbiota-gut-brain axis. Here's how it works:

1. The gut microbiome produces important messenger chemicals that influence brain function.
2. The gut is modulated by the enteric nervous system (ENS) that resides between the multi-layered walls of the digestive tract. The ENS is a crucial bridge between the microbes in the gut and various other systems in the body, including the brain.
3. The chemicals which the microbes produce can pass through the gut walls to interact with the ENS directly or stimulate other cells, releasing more substances that interact with the ENS.
4. Signals from the microbes are relayed via the ENS to the brain in different ways, such as via the bloodstream or nerve cells.
5. A significant communication channel between the gut and brain is the vagus nerve. This nerve connects the ENS to the central nervous system.
6. When the chemicals arrive at the brain, they're sent to different areas that impact various bodily processes.

This is a pretty basic explanation of an immensely complex communication system. The key idea to understand is that the gut and brain are in constant communication, via the microbiota-gut-brain axis, and they send signals back and forth that influence each other. To demonstrate this communication, think about when you see food that you think looks extremely tasty. Your brain will send your gut the message to get ready for food to arrive; you'll probably feel hunger pangs, and your mouth may even start watering. Similarly, when you're feeling anxious or stressed, you might experience gut-related symptoms such as stomach pain, nervous "butterflies", or nausea. Signals going in the opposite direction from gut to brain have symptoms that are a little more complex to detect, and we'll delve into that a little later in the chapter. For now, let's look at some ways your brain can affect your gut health.

YOUR BRAIN, YOUR GUT, AND STRESS

Stress is a physical, mental and emotional response to some-thing you perceive as a threat. Despite the bad rap stress has gotten over the years, it is actually natural and vital for human life. It is a natural response to potential threats and forms part of the fight-or-flight reaction that has been crucial to human survival in the past. Modern human beings, also known as homo sapiens, appeared around 300,000 years ago, long before livestock farming, agriculture, and human settlements arose (What Does It Mean To Be Human?, 2021). As such, our species started out as nomadic hunter-gather-ers, and our primitive means of protection still left us very much vulnerable to predators. Further still, things like natural disasters, including flooding and drought, also posed a real threat to our ancestors. Stress has long been the body's response to threats such as being attacked by animals, food scarcity, or natural disasters. In modern times, however, what we perceive as threatening has evolved drastically.

Some current threats can logically be linked to instinctual survival. For example:

- Employment insecurity or unemployment can feel like a threat to a person's survival because we need money to afford shelter, food, and more.
- Work stress or work performance stress similarly to the point above, causes worry about the ability to ensure survival through earning an income.
- Civil and political unrest or war will cause stress As well as concerns for one's safety directly due to being in a dangerous situation, there are concerns about the effect on the economy, commodity availability, employment, and other aspects of societal living, which potentially indirectly affects survival.

Those are just a few examples of how modern stressors can be linked to our survival instinct in an unimaginably different world from the one our ancestors inhabited. However, in this modern world we now have to deal with additional stressors that our ancestors did not. Modern stressors are uniquely a result of our societal advancement, including technology, social media, and societal expectations. For example, Studies have proven that life has become measurably more stressful in just the past 50 years, with lower adult stress levels and higher levels of wellbeing being reported in the 1990s compared to the 2010s (David et al., 2020).

A major contributor to modern-day stress is technology and

social media. People are more connected than ever before, and they are under pressure to appear to have the perfect life. While this stress isn't directly related to actual survival, it's a significant source of stress in modern life. That is only one example of current stressors that affect us daily but don't necessarily correlate to historic survival-related stressors. Ultimately, life has become more stressful in the past few decades. The brain is responsible for what is perceived as a threat or stressor, whether it's instinctive based on historical and intuitive survival mechanisms or learned through modern societal conditioning. Your brain decides what stresses you out and what doesn't. Therefore, the 'buck stops' at your brain. Regardless of what you know instinctually or have been conditioned to learn, your brain controls your stress response and, therefore, affects your gut health.

Before we deep dive into stress and how it affects your holistic wellbeing, it's important to distinguish between stress and anxiety. The two are often confused as the same thing, as symptoms can overlap. However, there is a fine line between stress, anxiety, and depression.

Stress, Anxiety, and Depression

Stress is usually a result of an external cause or trigger. Stressors can be short-term, such as an imminent work deadline that will pass, meaning the stress will dissipate. There are also long-term stressors, such as dealing with a chronic, incurable illness you have indefinitely. Stress typically results in symptoms such as irritability, muscle tension, fatigue, and digestive upset. Anxiety, however, is generally considered to be consistent, persistent, and excessive worry or fear. It doesn't necessarily have a particular reason for occurring and doesn't go away because if there is no reason, the reason cannot pass. The confusion between stress and anxiety is due to the similarity of the symptoms; The symptoms of anxiety mimic stress symptoms, including sleep issues, digestive upset, muscle tension, and irritability. The big difference is the source of the response. For stress, there is a discernible source, while for anxiety, there usually may not be a source. For example, stress may arise from being laid off. It goes away once you get a new job and a stable source of income. Anxiety would be having been laid off and having found new employment but still consistently worrying about financial security despite finding new, permanent employment and being financially secure. Both stress and anxiety can feed into depression.

Depression is a mood condition that can have many causes, from genetics to life circumstances. Two influential contributors to the development of depression are stress and anxiety.

- Studies have linked chronic stress, or prolonged periods of stress, with the increased risk of developing depression over time (Tafet & Nemeroff, 2015).
- While anxiety can often be a symptom of depression, research has also found a correlation between chronic anxiety disorders and a higher risk of developing depression (Sawchuk, 2017).

In the bigger picture, chronic stress or anxiety can lead to the development of depression, but depression can also give rise to stress and anxiety. The three states of emotional and mental distress can be symptoms of each other; they can also be contributing factors for each other. However, stress is of particular concern as, according to the World Health Organization (2023), people who experience unpleasant or adverse life events [i.e., experience stress] are at a higher risk and more likely to develop depression. In this way, stress, anxiety, and depression are linked, and all three can severely impact gut health.

How We Experience Stress

Stress can present itself in different ways.

- Physically: Symptoms include muscle tension, pain, aches, an increased heart rate, elevated blood pressure, digestive upset, headaches, fatigue, and other physical signs
- Mentally: Symptoms include memory issues, lack of concentration, anxiety, and loss of motivation are just a few of the mental signs of stress
- Behaviorally: Symptoms include a change in someone's regular habits, a change in appetite, the ditching of responsibilities or accountability, disturbed sleep, and changes in social interaction (such as social withdrawal)

- Emotionally: Symptoms include increased impulsivity, mood swings, prolonged sadness, irritability, listlessness

Types of Stress

Stress isn't equal. There are three different types of stress based on their frequency and duration. Each type of stress can manifest mentally, physically, emotionally, and behaviorally with similar symptoms, and you can experience more than one type of stress with overlapping symptoms at the same time. As confusing as this may sound, once you understand the different types of stress, you can figure out which ones you are experiencing and how to approach dealing with them.

Acute: Stress and its symptoms are short-lived and usually arise in response to a new or unexpected temporary situation. Examples of acute stress include being involved in a motor accident, getting a fright, or even having an enjoyable but thrilling experience such as riding a rollercoaster, or attaining a significant personal achievement. The mind, body, and emotions usually quickly equalize and return to normal once the "stressor" (or the 'trigger' of the stress) is over.

Acute episodic: This is very similar to acute stress, but it happens regularly instead of once in a while. It can result from regular acute stress from frequent stressful life events or working a high-pressure job. The critical difference between acute, acute episodic, and chronic stress is that there are short periods of reprieve from being in a state of acute stress response. Still, it's not enough to support proper recovery and return to equilibrium between acute stressor events, but the stress isn't always your companion all the time. The problem with acute episodic stress is that it can become so frequent that there is no reprieve anymore, and it becomes chronic. This occurs if there is continually one crisis after another.

Chronic: This is continual and consistent stress experienced over a prolonged period. Acute episodic stress can easily become chronic stress due to a convergence of circumstances. When you're suffering from chronic stress, you're likely to feel that stress is unending. This could be due to such reasons as living in a high-crime area, having constant relationship struggles, or experiencing frequent acute stress situations that don't offer you time to relax in between. This kind of stress is usually accompanied by a sense of inability to escape the situations causing the stress, feeling trapped; it is as if there is no "light at the end of the tunnel".

Symptoms by Stress Type

The symptoms of different kinds of stress can overlap, while some are specific to a particular form of stress. Here's how to recognize the symptoms of each kind of stress:

Acute:

- Anxiety
- Dilated pupils

- Elevated heart rate
- Emotional turbulence, or mood ups and downs
- Heavy/quick breathing
- Sleep disturbance
- Sweating

Acute episodic:

- Anger
- Higher blood pressure
- Feeling overwhelmed
- Headaches or migraines
- Irritability
- Muscle tension

Chronic:

- Anxiety or sometimes panic attacks
- Headaches or migraines
- Chronic muscle tension that may interfere with daily life
- Mental, physical, and emotional fatigue
- Sleep disturbances or insomnia
- Weight loss or gain

How Stress Affects Gut Health

You've probably already experienced the symptoms of stress on your gut before, but how does stress cause these issues?

Stress and its associated chemicals can alter gut bacteria populations, interfering with brain health and mental wellness. Often, populations of beneficial bacteria decline, leaving room for more non-beneficial bacteria (Foster, Rinaman, & Cryan, 2017). Some common symptoms of stress-related gut dysbiosis, or imbalance, include:

- Abdominal pain
- Bloating
- Change in stomach acidity
- Increased permeability of the gut lining
- Decreased mucous production
- Nausea
- Slower digestion
- Vomiting

Stress can impact gut health and set off a vicious cycle in which impaired gut health may affect how you experience stress. That is to say, due to the signaling link between the gut and brain, this change in the gut microbiome could also alter your psychological responses to stressors. Gut microbes interact with the hypothalamic-pituitary-adrenal axis or HPA axis. The HPA axis is a significant endocrine system that controls your stress response. When you're faced with a stressor, a structure in the brain called the hypothalamus is activated to release a hormone that signals your sympathetic nervous system to jump into action. This is how your fight-or-flight response is stimulated. This same hormone released by your hypothalamus also wakes up your pituitary gland, which, in turn, releases another hormone that sends a message to your adrenal glands to produce stress chemicals, such as adrenaline and cortisol (Tresca, 2022). Therefore, the communication between your gut and the HPA axis also has a further-reaching effect on the rest of the body via hormone production and release.

One of the results of this communication actually exacerbates your already unhappy gut by causing inflammation. When stressed, your body produces a natural stress hormone called cortisol. Cortisol is one of several glucocorticoids. These are steroid hormones that affect various bodily functions, including metabolism, and it's a natural part of your body's stress response. However, while it is a helpful hormone for managing stress, it can also become unhealthy. Stress isn't meant to be experienced for prolonged periods, and cortisol is intended to only be circulating for a short time until the stressor is dealt with or goes away. Chronic stress is the presence of persistent unhealthy stress levels over a long period, leading to consistently elevated cortisol levels. This can harm your gut health by causing inflammation, which disturbs the gut microbiome and the bacteria that live there. Stress can also increase the levels of harmful bacteria by impairing intestinal muscle function, impeding the ability of your gut to filter out those bacteria and thus adding to the inflammation.

Finally, stress, and its related inflammatory effect, also disrupts the communication flow along the microbiota-brain-gut-axis by affecting the vagus nerve. This nerve doesn't tolerate inflammation well. Chronic stress and the resulting systemic inflammation caused by higher-than-normal cortisol levels impairs the vagus nerve's ability to effectively pass messages between the gut and brain. When this communication highway doesn't work correctly, it's not only gut health that suffers, but your mental wellness too.

THE GUT HEALTH AND MENTAL WELLNESS CONNECTION

So far, we've discussed how the gut and brain communicate with each other, focusing on the role of the brain in this biochemical 'conversation'. The brain is a significant player in stress, anxiety, mood, emotions, and mental wellness difficulties such as depression, but it's not solely responsible for those things. The gastrointestinal tract also influences things that are typically considered to be the brain's responsibilities. An unhappy brain can lead to an unhappy gut, but the opposite is also true; an unhealthy gut can lead to an unhappy brain.

The leading cause of mental upset when your gut is unhealthy, comes down to neurotransmitters. Neurotransmitters are chemical signals sent between brain cells, and they're involved in numerous brain functions that affect the entire body. Serotonin is just one of dozens of neurotransmitters, but its impact is profound. It's commonly known as the body's "feel-good" hormone, but it also supports gut health by encouraging an optimum microbiome through regulating bowel function. This feel-good hormone influences your mental wellness by affecting your mood and emotions, and approximately 90% of it is produced in your gut (The Surprising Link Between Your Microbiome and Mental Health, n.d.).

Gut dysbiosis has been scientifically proven to impact mental or neurological conditions, such as depression and anxiety. More often than not, conditions like depression are linked with chemical imbalances in the brain, specifically related to serotonin. However, considering the gut's role in producing the vast majority of the body's serotonin, depression may really be caused by an imbalance in your gut, resulting in a disruption in serotonin production. Additionally, inflammation in the gut might be a contributing factor to anxiety, as it's been shown to increase the release of chemicals that have been directly linked to anxiety (Bose, 2023).

WHAT'S NEXT?

Gut health and mental wellness are inextricably connected through the gut-brain axis. When one is troubled, the other suffers as well. This means that your approach to a healthy lifestyle must be holistic; it should entail looking after both your physical and mental wellness. The good news about improving your physical health is that many traditional concepts of a healthy lifestyle support gut and mental health, but we want to delve deeper into overall wellness. To truly support your overall wellness, you need to discover strategies that nourish your mental wellbeing by reducing stress, increasing positivity, alleviating anxiety, and relieving or preventing depression. In the four-part guide to come, we'll tackle the four pillars of a gut-brain-healthy lifestyle: mindfulness, nutrition, physical activity, and mental and emotional wellbeing. You can apply the knowledge and strategies provided in a way that suits you best, focusing on one part of the guide at a time or implementing different principles simultaneously. The key is to actively invest in improving and maintaining your gut and mental health in easy steps that anybody can take.

2

PART 1: MINDFULLY SUPPORTING GUT HEALTH AND MENTAL WELLNESS

Mindfulness is a topic that has been gaining popularity and traction as society opens its collective mind to teachings and philosophies from different cultures around the globe. So, you may have heard about it, but what does it really mean? Mindfulness is the ability to be 100% aware and present in the moment. This means having full awareness of oneself physically, mentally, and emotionally, as well as of the environment and situation. Its awareness of one's own actions, thoughts, and emotions while not becoming overwhelmed or overreacting to what is happening in the present moment.

Breaking it down further, the practice of mindfulness has its origins in the East and is referenced in Buddhist scriptures. These scriptures describe mindfulness as a way to help view life and ourselves with greater clarity and use that clarity to make wiser choices and respond better to the things that happen. Mindfulness practices have their origins in ancient Chinese medicine, but they have made the leap into modern society, where science now supports the various mental and physical benefits (Sutton, 2019).

MINDFULNESS AND THE BRAIN

We've already explored how the gut and brain are inextricably linked and affect each other. Mindfulness can effectively enhance emotional regulation, reduce stress, and cultivate mental positivity. These benefits ultimately influence gut health; a healthier mental state supports a healthier gut. So, let's look at how it specifically affects the brain.

- **Frontal cortex:** Also called the frontal lobe, this is the front part of your brain, and it's in charge of motor control, abstract thinking, judgment, socially appropriate behavior, and creativity. Consistent mindfulness practices have been shown to gradually improve efficacy of the frontal cortex. The increased efficacy improves the ability to think rationally, plan ahead, control impulses, and be aware of and control emotions.
- **Social neural circuitry:** Neural circuitry refers to the nerve cell networks within the brain that carry messages to different areas. When activated, these neural messengers are responsible for cognitive and physiological responses. Social neural circuits send messages to the parts of the brain governing social

interaction. Mindfulness is associated with increased density of gray matter in the parts of the brain related to social interaction, greater relationship satisfaction, and maintaining healthy relationships.

- **Amygdala:** The amygdala is a small but powerful structure in your brain. Its main job is processing emotions and linking those feelings to various other functions, such as the senses, learning, and memory. It plays a huge role in survival by controlling fear and anxiety. The more active the amygdala is, the more likely you are to experience fear and anxiety. Mindfulness is associated with lower activity levels in this part of the brain, which is linked to less anxiety and increased feelings of calm and mental wellness.

- **Anterior cingulate cortex:** This is a section of the brain in charge of many different functions, including how emotions are expressed, regulating mood, and the ability to focus attention. Mindfulness has been found to stimulate the anterior cingulate cortex, which can improve attention, emotional regulation, and motivation.

(Linder, 2019)

Now that you know how mindfulness benefits your brain to enhance mental wellness and in turn, gut health, it's time to discover some valuable techniques.

MINDFULNESS TECHNIQUES

Understanding how mindfulness works isn't going to help much if the understanding is not put into practice, just as understanding how diet and exercise improve your health doesn't actually improve your health. It's crucial to practice mindfulness to tap into the many benefits it offers. It's also not something you'll learn by doing it once or twice. It's a skill that has to be learned and practiced regularly to be effective, and, like learning to play a sport or an instrument, one can improve at the skill.

Learning any new skill can come with difficulties. Some people find it challenging to learn and practice mindfulness for various reasons. Some common obstacles to learning and practicing mindfulness techniques include:

- **Lack of time:** It's a misconception that you must spend a large chunk of your day practicing mindfulness or meditation to improve at it and for it to become more effective. All you need is as little as 10 minutes per day.
- **Discomfort:** When you picture someone meditating, you probably come up with the stereotypical image of someone sitting cross-legged in the lotus position on the ground. Mindfulness practice doesn't have to be uncomfortable, and you can do it in a position that works for you or even try moving mindfulness meditations.
- **Intrusive thoughts:** Your mind is always thinking,

and trying to stop and completely empty your mind is virtually impossible. Experiencing a noisy mind and intrusive thoughts during mindfulness or meditation is normal. What different techniques will teach you is not to let these thoughts hijack your attention and run away with you.

- **Inability to see the benefit:** As with any skill, it takes time, practice, and consistency to reap the rewards of mindfulness. You cannot pick up a musical instrument for the first time and expect to play flawlessly, but you will see improvements over time. You aren't likely to immediately see the benefits of mindfulness. It can take weeks. Patience and consistency are vital for learning to practice techniques effectively and start seeing the results.

- **Distractions:** Sounds and sights of the world around you will always be there. The stillness and quiet you seek come from inside and don't require you to be in a soundless, distraction-free environment. The more you practice mindfulness, the less often any distractions will draw your attention.

- **Self-doubt:** This is a big obstacle for many who try to practice mindfulness or meditation. The problem is the notion that there is a right or wrong way to do it or that one technique should work for everyone. These misconceptions may leave you feeling that you just can't get a technique right or to be effective. If you're struggling with one technique, try another. Find the one that works best for you.

Before You Start

Before you start learning mindfulness, grab a pen and a piece of paper and answer a few questions. Physically writing down your answers can be a powerful way to solidify your intentions instead of simply answering in your head. It's a way of grounding you in the moment and, as such, can even be seen as your very first mindfulness practice. As you answer the questions, focus on and be mindful of your commitment to your mindfulness journey and your intentions.

Why do you want to learn mindfulness? Putting in the time and effort necessary to learn a new skill is usually driven by a desire for specific outcomes. Think about the benefits of mindfulness and pick out those which motivate you to become more mindful. You may want to cultivate mental calm, emotional regulation, self-acceptance, better relationships, psychological positivity, or any number of other reasons.

What are some of your strengths? There are often aspects of ourselves we want to improve on or things we want to change. However, it's vital to recognize our strengths or positive qualities. Self-improvement cannot be achieved from a place of negativity or self-deprecation. It's not a good idea to focus only on what we want to improve. Make a list of your core strengths. If you have difficulty seeing the good in yourself, think about what your best friend or someone close to you would say they value about you.

When will you practice mindfulness techniques? Committing to consistently practicing mindfulness techniques is often a considerable challenge. Decide when the best time would be for you to practice. Some people find it easier just before bed, or first thing in the morning. Some find another time to practice, when they are less likely to be interrupted. There will always be some unforeseen circumstances which will mean you cannot practice mindfulness at your chosen time, but committing to a consistent routine practice time will help you.

Where will you practice mindfulness techniques? Picking a space to practice in can make or break your experience. Try to find somewhere separate from your usual and dominant distractions, such as other people, technology, or entertainment. Ensure where you practice is comfortable, inviting, feels safe, and encourages mental and emotional calm.

Body Scan

Performing a body scan encourages you to become in tune with the physical sensations of your body. This technique can reduce stress and anxiety. It also helps the practitioner to become more comfortable with various bodily sensations, and the various emotions linked to them. To perform a body scan of yourself, do the following:

- Get into a comfortable position, lying down, sitting, or standing.
- Close your eyes and focus on your breath.
- Bring attention to any part of your body. This can be

your foot, or hand, or the top of your head. I can be anywhere you'd like to begin.

- Focus on that body part, breathing slowly and deeply, and become aware of any unusual sensations.
- Spend up to a minute observing the sensations.
- Acknowledge the sensations and any emotions they may evoke.
- Accept the emotions that may arise without judging them, and without judging yourself for having them. Accept them without allowing them to overwhelm you.
- Continue breathing deeply and slowly, imagining any unpleasant sensations ebbing away with each exhalation.
- After a few breaths, release focus on that particular body part as you exhale and refocus on another body part as you inhale.
- Repeat the body scan across your entire body in any order that feels right to you until you've spent time being aware of every area.
- If your thoughts wander astray, gently bring your awareness and focus back to where you are in the body scan.
- Once you've completed the body scan, focus on your breath before you end the session.

Breathing Exercises

Breathing exercises are useful to reduce both stress and anxiety by shifting your attention from your thoughts and emotions to your breath. This can de-escalate negative thoughts and emotions before they become overwhelming and thus it can give you time to react in a calmer way to whatever caused them. Alternatively, breathing exercises can be used to create a sense of calm, such as before sleep. Three popular techniques are easy to practice and only take a few minutes: they are called Dirga Pranayama, Sam Vritti Pranayama (with Antara Kumbhaka and Bahya Kumbhaka), and Nadi Shodhana Pranayama.

Dirga Pranayama

Also called diaphragm breathing, this technique is a proven stress and anxiety reduction strategy that also boosts higher cognitive functions, such as awareness, memory, and language, and positively impacts the nervous system (Majsiak & Young, 2022).

- Get into a comfortable position. You could be lying down, sitting, or standing. Then place one hand gently on your abdomen.
- Take a few regular deep breaths, bringing awareness to your breath when it is entering and leaving your body.
- When you're ready to begin, focus on breathing into your abdomen.
- Envision your breath flowing below your chest and filling your abdomen like a balloon as your ribs expand.

- Your ribs will expand when you inhale, but by breathing into your abdomen, your shoulders and chest should only move minimally.
- As you exhale, envision your stomach deflating and your navel being drawn in toward your spine.
- Perform 3-5 or up to 10 deep diaphragm breaths.

Sama Vritti Pranayama with Antara Kumbhaka and Bahya Kumbhaka

This technique is also referred to as box breathing or '4-7-8 breathing'. It's a kind of intermittent breathing pattern based on counting up to certain numbers. It has been shown to reduce anxiety, depression, and breathlessness (Majsiak & Young, 2022). Many different counting patterns can be used other than 4-7-8, such as 4-4-4. However, it's essential to set your own pattern when you start out with this technique. Begin with a low number that is high enough to slow your breathing down but isn't uncomfortable. A good starting point is 3-4 seconds. Each count is 1-second long. You can increase or change the numbers in your pattern as you get more comfortable.

- Sit in a comfortable, relaxed position.
- Exhale deeply through your mouth, pushing all the air out of your lungs.
- Close your mouth and inhale through your nose, drawing your breath into your abdomen, counting to your desired number as you breathe deeply to fill your lungs.

- Hold your breath as you count to your desired number.
- Exhale deeply through your mouth as you count to your desired number, emptying your lungs.
- For example, to practice a '4-4-4' counting pattern, do these three steps: inhale for a count of 4, or 4 seconds. Hold your breath for 4 seconds. Exhale for 4 seconds.
- Perform this intermittent breathing pattern 3-7 times.

Important note: Breathing exercises may cause light headedness. It's important to practice them in a safe environment where you're not likely to harm yourself or others if you do begin to feel light headed. For example, never perform breathing exercises while driving a vehicle or operating machinery..

Nadi Shodhana Pranayama

You may hear this technique called alternate-nostril yoga breathing. It's excellent for reducing stress and, specifically, blood pressure. Studies have revealed that this breathing technique, used twice daily for 10 minutes per session, effectively improves heart rate and lowers blood pressure (Majsiak & Young, 2022).

- Sit in a comfortable, relaxed position.

- Place your right hand on your right knee and press your left thumb gently against your left nostril to close it.
- Slowly inhale through your right nostril.
- Release your left nostril and gently press your right nostril closed with your left ring finger.
- Hold your breath for a second or two.
- Exhale slowly through your left nostril.
- Inhale slowly through your left nostril.
- Release your right nostril and gently press your left nostril closed with your left thumb again.
- Hold your breath for a second or two.
- Exhale slowly through your right nostril.
- Repeat 5-10 times or between 10.

Mindful Eating

In today's world, mealtimes have become sorely neglected. It's more common to rush through a meal or eat while multi-tasking to save time. When meals become a sit-down affair, there are usually many distractions, such as TV or mobile devices. This culture of rushed or distracted mealtimes has encouraged "mindless" eating. How often do you eat more than you realize or finish your meal without realizing it?

Mindfulness can be practiced in many aspects of your life, including your relationship with food. You can focus your awareness on the moment while grocery shopping, preparing meals, serving food, and eating. Paying attention to your senses, thoughts, emotions, and physical sensations can help you improve your relationship with food and make adopting healthier eating habits easier.

Benefits of Mindful Eating

- **Stress relief:** Taking time out of your day to slow down, eat slowly, focus on your meal, and enjoy your food can help ease anxiety and reduce stress.
- **Healthier relationships with food:** Mindful eating isn't just about consuming food or beverages but also about noticing hunger cues, cravings, and noticing how you feel when you eat. Becoming in tune with your eating habits provides the opportunity to take a closer look at your relationship with food and may allow you to make changes if you notice unwanted tendencies.
- **Portion control:** Taking time to eat slowly and noticing satiation cues instead of distractedly wolfing down your food can help you eat less.
- **Digestion:** Eating slower is better for digestion, and improved digestion is healthier for your gut.
- **Healthy choices:** Often, less healthy options may leave you feeling bloated, result in digestive discomfort, cause a blood sugar spike and crash, or even make you feel guilty. By focusing on how different foods make you feel during and after eating

them, you can start to intuitively make healthier choices.

- **Pleasure:** Eating is usually an inherently pleasant experience, especially when you consume foods you like. Slowing down and opening your awareness to the delightful flavors, smells, textures, emotions, and physical sensations allows you to extract every ounce of pleasure from mealtimes.

How to Eat Mindfully

- Take a few deep breaths to slow down and shift your focus to the groceries you're shopping for, to the preparation of the meal, and to the moment when eating the food.
- Use all your senses while preparing and eating a meal. Take in the colors, shapes, and textures of different food items. Concentrate on both how they feel as they are being prepared, and what they smell like. Listen to how they sound as they are being prepared and cooked. Appreciate the visual appeal of the plated food and the aromas. Enjoy how the food feels and tastes in your mouth as you eat. You can even try to identify individual flavors and ingredients by their aroma and taste.
- Maintain mindfulness of your body while eating. Ensure you sit in a comfortable, relaxed position with good posture. Focus on releasing any tension

you might feel in your muscles in order to properly relax.

- Maintain mindfulness throughout your meal. Avoid allowing environmental distractions to take your attention away from what you are doing.
- Put your utensils down regularly or even between bites. This helps slow you down and avoids rushing. Eating slowly is vital for mindful eating.
- Be grateful. Practicing a little gratitude for the food you have and where it came from can have an emotionally positive impact.
- Pay attention to your hunger. You should eat when receiving reasonable hunger cues and avoid skipping meals. If you eat when you are ravenous due to skipping meals or waiting too long, you could rush through the meal or overeat. Identify whether you are actually hungry or merely tempted to have a meal or snack because others are eating and you feel you are expected to join in, or because you're bored, or frustrated, or unhappy, for example.
- Pay attention to your body and cravings. Cravings can be your body telling you it's nutritionally lacking something or that you need to examine your emotions, which could be nudging you to crave specific kinds of food.
- Experiment with food. Try different kinds of food, swapping ingredients, or even removing or limiting foods or ingredients. Pay attention to how including new foods or excluding some potentially

problematic foods makes you feel after your meals. Try to identify foods that make your body feel nourished and good, and also identify those that don't. This way, you can avoid foods that don't agree with you. Be aware not to eliminate whole food groups without either consulting your medical doctor first. If you want to introduce new ingredients or foods, test them in small quantities first to see if you have any intolerances. If you have previously experienced intolerances or have close family members with known allergies or intolerances to new ingredients you want to introduce, first consult your doctor about the safety of introducing these ingredients and how to safely go about including them.

Use a Hunger Scale

You may be wondering why you need a scale to compare your hunger. If you've spent a lot of time skipping meals, rushing through eating, or acting on mental or emotional hunger signals, you may need to be more in tune with your body. A hunger-satiety scale, like the one below, can help you more effectively listen to and follow your body's cues, in order to avoid waiting till you're overly hungry, overeating, or eating for the wrong reasons. Here is the scale:

1. Starving, feeling weak or faint, lacking energy
2. Really hungry, feeling a little light-headed or dizzy, feeling tired and listless

3. Hungry, uncomfortable hunger pangs, feeling irritable, unable to concentrate.
4. Hungry, stomach growling, otherwise feeling fine
5. Hunger is starting to set in
6. Satisfied, but able to eat a little bit more
7. Stomach feels full, but you're not uncomfortable
8. Stomach feels overfull and slightly uncomfortable
9. Stomach feels stuffed and very uncomfortable
10. Stomach feels fit to burst and may be painful, and you're likely to feel sick

Aim to stay in the 4-7 range, which means you're not too hungry nor too full. When you reach 3, stop whatever you are doing to make time to eat. You're less likely to make healthy choices or eat mindfully when you're overly hungry. You're also more at risk of rushing and eating too much before you notice your stomach getting full. When you reach 6, stop eating and wait 15-20 minutes. This gives your brain time to register that your stomach is full, and you'll likely not want to eat anymore.

TIPS FOR INCORPORATING MINDFULNESS DAILY

Mindfulness requires consistency to deliver results. You can't practice it once and hope to be rewarded. Even once a week isn't often enough for mindfulness to be effective. It should become a part of your everyday life. The more you practice, the sooner you'll get better at it and the quicker you'll start experiencing the benefits. Use the following tips to incorporate mindfulness into your daily routine.

Check-in with yourself: Your body keeps functioning despite how busy your day gets. You don't stop breathing, and your heart doesn't stop beating just because you're not focused on it. This can lend itself to 'tuning out' or failing to notice a variety of bodily sensations that could relay vital messages to you. Take some time daily to pay attention to how your body feels, especially any unpleasant sensations such as muscle tension, pain, or fatigue. Your body is sending you signals which you can use to learn how to better care for your physical and mental wellbeing.

Be grateful: Taking a few moments to focus on what you are thankful for at the moment helps bring your awareness back to the present and infuse positivity into your day. This is especially helpful for easing anxiety and stress if you find yourself worrying about something in the future or fixated on something from the past. Gratitude can help break the cycle, return you to the present moment, and allow you to continue with a less anxious and more positive attitude.

Tune into your senses: Tuning into your senses is a simple but effective way to focus on the present and ground yourself in the moment you're living in. It's handy if you feel stressed, anxious, or overwhelmed. Stop what you are doing and spend a few moments observing your surroundings. Pick a few things you can see, hear, smell, touch, and taste. If you have time to spare, spend time noticing what's happening around you and what others are doing.

Listen actively: This guide discusses active listening in-depth in Part 4. At least once a day, commit to practicing the principles of active listening. Over time, it'll be easier to apply the principles to all your conversations. Remember to take note of how active listening improves your communication with others.

Take advantage of situations to practice mindfulness: There are plenty of daily opportunities. You just have to take advantage of them. These situations include:

- Walking: While you're walking, turn your attention to your bodily sensations. Notice how your clothes feel and move, how your feet feel as they make contact with the ground, how your arms feel and swing, how your hips move and rotate, and any other body sensations you become aware of. Focus on maintaining good posture while you're walking.
- Eating: Try to practice mindful eating during meals.
- Showering or bathing: Open your awareness to all the physical sensations of showering or bathing. Notice the temperature of the water, the steam rising, the sensation of the soap suds or body wash, how your sponge feels as you run it over your skin, or the scent of the soap, for example.
- Waiting: When you realize you have to wait, become aware of yourself. Notice any emotions you may feel, such as frustration, anger, irritation, and thoughts about waiting. Don't focus on those emotions or

thoughts. Observe them without judgment and let them go. Shift your focus to your body and pay attention to body's sensations and your breath, drawing attention away from your emotions and thoughts.

- Social interactions: When interacting with someone else, ground yourself in the interaction and focus your attention on the other person. Engage in active listening to prevent your mind from wandering away from the interaction. Focus on the other person's non-verbal communication, such as body language and tone of voice. Picking up on non-verbal cues can help you better determine how to act and react to foster better relationships.

TRACK YOUR MINDFULNESS JOURNEY

It cannot be stressed enough that mindfulness is a skill. Everyone is inherently able to be mindful, but that doesn't mean they'll be good at it. Effective mindfulness takes practice, and it can take a while before improvements or benefits are noticed. Tracking your journey is a valuable way to truly notice all the changes and improvements you make along the way, especially when they're small and easily overlooked.

After each mindfulness exercise, record the following information:

- The date and time of the exercise
- What exercise you did

- Your impressions of the experience

Record your practice session immediately after you've finished so you remember all the details. The impressions of your practice session can include:

- Thoughts that came up during the exercise
- Emotions that you felt
- Physical sensations you experienced
- How the practice felt: if it was easy, difficult, uncomfortable, or relaxing, for example
- Distractions that came up and how you responded to them

Keeping a mindfulness tracking journal can provide insights into yourself and your journey. You can look back on past practice experiences and compare them with recent ones to see, for example, how you are progressing, or where you may be struggling, or where you're improving, or what kinds of practices work best for you, or the times and places that make practices easier.

WHAT'S NEXT?

Mindfulness is a powerful and effective strategy for improving mental wellness in a variety of ways. Mindfulness techniques can improve relationships, stress management, self-care, improved eating habits, and mental positivity. Adding mindfulness to your day doesn't have to take up a large chunk of time, and you can practice simple methods almost anywhere and at virtually any time. You'll need to be patient with yourself and with the process, though. Like any other healthy habit, it takes a while of consistent practice to develop mindfulness as a skill. Then you will start seeing the benefits of the commitment to mastering it. One of the aspects of mindfulness we've covered is mindful eating. Learning to eat more mindfully lays the foundation for another pillar of overall gut-brain health: nutrition. Eating a healthy, balanced diet is commonly accepted to support general wellbeing, but it extends beyond just giving your body what it needs to function optimally. In the next part of this guide, we'll explore how nutrition can affect your gut and mental health, as well as foods that are good for your gut and brain, and we will explore strategies to make it easy to adopt a more nutritious diet.

3

PART 2: NUTRITIONALLY SUPPORTING GUT HEALTH AND MENTAL WELLNESS

The phrase "you are what you eat" is usually an insult or criticism aimed at either shaming people for their food choices or guilting them into eating more healthily. However, this concept isn't too far off the mark when it comes to the power of nutrition on the body and mind. Every cell in the body needs nutrients to function optimally. When those nutrients aren't available, cells, tissues, and systems can't perform as they should, and it begins to show. Some nutritional deficiencies have clearly apparent symptoms, such as a shortage of vitamin C resulting in scurvy or tearing the sides of the mouth. Other deficiencies may cause lackluster hair, brittle nails, or other evidently visible signs that your body isn't getting what it needs for your diet. On the other hand, other symptoms of nutrient shortages are harder to attribute to an imbalance in your diet, such as fatigue, digestive problems, brain fog, or mood swings.

What you put into your body, or what you don't, dramatically affects both physical and mental health, pointing to the truth that what you eat contributes significantly to who you are. In this chapter, we will explore the vital role of nutrition in gut health and mental wellness and how different nutrients can positively or negatively affect both.

THE ROLE OF NUTRITION IN GUT HEALTH

It's widely accepted that diet affects your general physical health and has been linked to either an increase or decrease in chronic disease risk. However, diet doesn't just affect your health in the most popularly publicized ways, such as influencing blood pressure, cholesterol, insulin sensitivity, and the cardiovascular system. It also impacts your gut and the bacteria that call this part of your body home.

Research has suggested that what you eat affects your gut bacteria populations and how much beneficial or detrimental bacteria inhabit this microbiome. This is understandable since those bacteria feed off your food, and some will flourish more substantially on certain foods. Science indicates that diet can be a key factor in improving the diversity of bacteria species and the stability of your gut health (Leeming et al., 2019).

That being said, how does nutrition affect these microscopic organisms that share your body?

Carbohydrates

Carbohydrates (or 'carbs') are a staple part of any balanced diet and are found in many foods, from bread to pasta to starchy vegetables. Carbs make up the primary source of energy and carbon for gut microbes. Aside from providing them with energy, carbohydrates affect gut microbes and the environment they inhabit in the following ways:

Complex carbs are rich in fiber, particularly the insoluble kind that doesn't get fully digested on its way through your system. This fiber aids gastrointestinal health and function by creating bulk, which absorbs water. As a result, toxins are diluted, digestion is made more efficient, and the whole process is sped up. Removing toxins and keeping the movement of food through the gut helps maintain a healthy environment for gut bacteria.

Fiber-rich carbs improve gut health by stimulating fermentation, which, in turn, encourages an increase in bacteria populations. Some bacteria in the gut feed on this fiber, and the metabolites, or substances created by their digestion of the fiber, are a source of energy for other bacteria. The more fiber there is, the more fiber-eating bacteria are supported. The more fiber-eating bacteria there are, the more energy-providing metabolites there are to feed larger populations of other bacteria species.

So far, the focus has been on complex carbohydrates. All carbohydrates are broken down into sugar, but simple carbs are more easily digested and contain higher sugar concentrations. These carbs are not good for your gut health as diets high in sugar can threaten gut microbiome health. Studies have found that a high-sugar diet is linked to an increased risk of colitis. Diets rich in sugar and simple carbs tend to increase gut lining permeability. When the gut lining is more permeable, toxins and microbes that should remain in the gut can escape and run amok in the rest of your body. Increased gut permeability has been linked to numerous inflammatory diseases, including inflammatory bowel disease, chronic kidney disease, and even chronic heart failure. However, that's not all. Your mental health can also take a knock if your gut allows unwanted microbes to exit, and gut permeability has even been associated with depression (Fukui & Kashihara, 2016).

Fats

Contrary to what popular dieting misconceptions would have you think, fat is a vital part of a healthy diet and is necessary for various bodily functions. There are different kinds, and not all are good for you. Some of the most well-known pitfalls of a high-fat diet are cardiovascular disease, hypertension, and elevated cholesterol levels. However, you may not realize how excess fat in your diet can cause gut dysbiosis.

Research has found that diets rich in fats, specifically trans and saturated fats, may contribute to chronic systemic inflammation and to increased risk of metabolic diseases. It's suspected that high-fat diets alter the bacterial composition within the gut, increase gut permeability, and damage the mucus layer. All three of these potential side effects likely contribute to problems with immune issues, as it has been found that fatty diets are linked to an increase in an immune-triggering compound called LPS. Lipopolysaccharide, or LPS, is a significant cell membrane component of some bacteria, but having an excess that escapes the gut and goes into circulation triggers pro-inflammatory immune responses throughout the body (Conlon & Bird, 2014).

The good news is that unsaturated fats, mainly monounsaturated fatty acids, have been linked to increased gut bacteria diversity for a healthier gut, but that's not all. Medium-chain fatty acids, found in both unsaturated and saturated fat, have been shown to encourage balance between microbial populations and improve the gut barrier's health and integrity (Bhowmik, 2023).

Protein

Most of the time, when someone mentions protein, you're probably thinking of steak, fish, chicken, lamb chops, and other sources of animal-based protein. Animal protein may be the most commonly recognized form of protein, but it's not the only one. Plants offer us protein as well. However, not all protein is created equal, and some sources are healthier than others. Plants offer healthier protein than animals in the battle between animal and plant proteins.

Research has discovered that diets rich in animal proteins can be harmful to your gut bacteria populations and that diets rich in plant proteins can benefit them. Consuming lots of animal proteins may increase the number of anaerobic bile-tolerant bacteria. This population boom is associated with higher levels of a compound linked to a greater risk of developing cardiovascular disease. Eating more animal protein is also associated with larger populations of sulfate-reducing bacteria which are linked to there being increased inflammation in the gut.

Consuming more plant proteins is associated with an increase in good gut bacteria while simultaneously decreasing populations of harmful gut bacteria. Specifically, eating more pulses or legumes is reported to positively impact gut microbes by reducing inflammation and helping to maintain beneficial stability in the environment the microbes call home (Bhowmik, 2023).

Food Additives

Additives have been in the negative limelight for quite some time. While some have been deemed bad and to be avoided, others are still being used and consumed every day. Additives are used for all sorts of reasons, from enhancing flavor to prolonging the shelf life of processed foods. The more heavily a food item is processed, the more additives it's likely to contain.

Emerging science is now making a case for minimizing processed foods and the amount of additives you're eating because of the potential links to health issues. Pre-clinical research suggests that consuming more food additives over a long period may contribute to developing or worsening metabolic syndrome, intestinal inflammation, various cancers, and colitis (Laudisi, Stolfi & Monteleone, 2019).

THE IMPACT OF NUTRITION ON MENTAL WELLNESS

It can often be easier to understand how nutrition affects the physical body rather than the mind, especially because it's something many are taught from a young age. As kids, many people are taught which foods are healthy and which are considered less healthy, and they're encouraged to make choices that will support their physical health. The impact of diet on the body in terms of chronic diseases is also widely publicized across various mediums such as the internet, magazines, health books, and even pamphlets. However, the influence nutrition has on mental wellness is often over-looked, and you may even come across the misconception that mental wellness is all in the mind. It's not. Mental wellness is affected by a myriad of factors, including nutrition. What you eat can affect your brain's physical makeup, cognition, and the chemicals needed to regulate mental function. This has serious implications for your mental wellness, including risk factors for anxiety, depression, and mood stability.

Diet and Your Brain

Your body derives everything it needs to create cells, fuel them with energy, and keep them healthy and functioning properly. Your brain is no exception. Without the correct nutrition, your brain's physical structure and functioning may be negatively affected. This influences cognitive processes as well as mood and emotion.

For example, numerous studies have shown that excessive consumption of refined sugars has a toxic effect on the brain due to the stress it places on the pancreas. Additionally, the sudden drop in blood sugar, associated with increased insulin production in response to a blood sugar spike, takes its toll. When blood sugar suddenly dips, cortisol and glucagon levels rise. These autonomic neurotransmitters are responsible for the associated increase in anxiety, irritability, and hunger that follows such a blood sugar drop. They're also attributed to aggravating the symptoms of different mood disorders and depression (Thomas, 2022).

Aside from unhealthy diets often increasing the amount of harmful substances in our bodies, they're also usually deficient in crucial nutrients. Micronutrients might be needed only in small amounts, but they're powerful and essential for a healthy body and mind. When you're not getting enough of each kind of nutrient, especially folate, cobalamin, and zinc, you could be at a higher risk of developing a mood disorder. Nutritional deficiencies have been linked to several symptoms of not only depression but also irritability and cognitive-decline disorders like dementia (Thomas, 2022).

Finally, let's look at how fat affects your brain. Some healthy fats, like the omega-3 fatty acids in fatty fish, have anti-inflammatory influences. These same inflammation-fighting fats are used to form essential parts of the membranes of brain cells and play key roles in various processes in the brain. When the brain doesn't get enough of them, brain cell structure and neurological processes are affected.

A GUT-HEALTHY DIET

Understanding the impact of nutrition on gut health and mental wellness is the first step toward changing your eating habits to transform your life. To make those changes, the following question to ask is, "What is a gut-healthy diet?"

The truth is there is no specific "gut-health diet" in the sense of a rigidly structured guideline as you would find with, for instance, the keto or Atkins diets. There are foods you are encouraged to include in your diet and foods you're warned about steering clear of or minimizing, but there's nothing you absolutely *must* include or cut out completely. Instead, a gut-healthy diet is a relatively broad concept that emphasizes certain practices:

- Food diversity
- Nutritionally dense foods
- Limiting foods that could be harmful to your gut
- Including gut-health superfoods
- Nutritional balance

As such, a gut-healthy diet offers much freedom to eat foods you enjoy, indulge in limited amounts of unhealthy foods, and eat intuitively. You don't have to follow any specific diet if you don't want to, but there is one diet that you could use as a fantastic guideline. The Mediterranean diet is considered one of the healthiest diets, if not *the* healthiest diet, in the world.

Research backs up the health claims of the Mediterranean diet or Mediterranean-style eating habits. Some health benefits associated with this diet include scaling back the risk of chronic diseases such as metabolic syndrome, cardiovascular disease, and several cancers, among other health conditions. It's also proven beneficial for your gut microbiome by improving regulation and microbe diversity. These benefits are attributed to the high amounts of unsaturated fatty acids, fiber, polyphenols, and antioxidants provided in the staple foods of the diet (Nagpal et al., 2019).

Many of the beneficial compounds in the Med diet come from plant sources. It's considered a plant-based diet. In modern society that has seen a rise in the popularity of veganism and the associated avoidance of eating animal products, and sometimes the mention of a "plant-based diet" brings a skewed picture to mind. 'Plant-based' doesn't mean a diet is strictly vegetarian or vegan. It just means that staple foods come from plants, emphasizing fruit, vegetables, grains, and other plant-derived foods. At the same time, animal protein and products are consumed in moderation or limited. Research is discovering that emphasizing plant foods, like the Mediterranean diet, increases gut bacteria diversity while boosting good microbe population numbers (Sidhu et al., 2023).

Another substantial positive the Med diet has going for it, in terms of supporting gut health, is the encouragement of dietary diversity. Not only does this expose you to a world of different flavors, textures, smells, and dishes. It's also crucial for improving the diversity of your gut bacteria. Different types of bacteria feed on different nutrients. When you restrict your diet to eating only a limited selection of foods, you're not providing your gut microbiome with food to support various species of bacteria. The more microbial diversity your gut supports, the greater your beneficial bacteria populations. This improves overall health and makes your gut ecosystem more adaptable to disturbances.

Finally, a gut-healthy diet may not just be about what you eat but also when you eat. Many diet-related factors, such as nutrition and maintaining a healthy weight, can influence gut health. An aspect that may play a role in improving or maintaining gut health is when you plan your meals. Time-restricted eating habits may contribute to increased gut microbe diversity for improved intestinal health. The more diverse the populations of your internal microbes, the more beneficial they are to your physical and mental wellness.

In our book, *Intermittent Fasting for Women,* we discuss the principles of intermittent fasting and explore the many ways anybody can adopt a time-restricted eating regime. If you think intermittent fasting is something you'd like to try in conjunction with the practices in this guide to improve your gut health, find *Intermittent Fasting for Women: A Guide to Creating a Sustainable, Long-Term Lifestyle for Weight Loss and Better Health! Includes*

How to Start, 16:8, 5:2, OMAD, Fast 800, ADM, Warrior, and Fast 5! on Amazon and get reading! P.S. Don't let the title fool you. The fasting strategies and benefits outlined in the book are just as applicable for men as they are for women!

FOODS THAT PROMOTE GUT HEALTH

So far, we've established that a diverse plant-based diet rich in nutrient-dense foods and healthy fatty acids is what you need to embrace to improve gut health through diet. While that gives you a tremendous amount of freedom as far as food choices go, it doesn't really tell you if there's anything specific you can eat to support your gut. Two main categories of foods promote gut health are prebiotics and probiotics.

Prebiotics

Prebiotics are substances found in plant-based foods that feed your beneficial gut bacteria. They specifically encourage the maintenance of healthy, good microbe populations. Prebiotics are fiber, but it's important to note that not all fiber is prebiotic. For example, the fiber from apples is prebiotic, but the fiber in white bread is not.

Increasing your intake of prebiotics provides more food to sustain more significant numbers of healthy gut bacteria, improve their health, and increase their survival in the gastrointestinal tract. In turn, these bacteria metabolize the prebiotic fiber and produce byproducts that benefit you by improving digestion, aiding nutrient absorption, and boosting immune function.

Fermentable oligosaccharides, disaccharides, monosaccharides, and polyols, also known as FODMAPs, are the richest sources of prebiotics. These indigestible fibers are fermented by certain microbes. As such, eating foods containing these substances could leave you with some natural fermentation side effects, like bloating and gas. Individuals dealing with irritable bowel syndrome (IBS) may experience discomfort from these symptoms. When adding prebiotic foods to your diet, opt for low-FODMAP items instead of those with higher concentrations so you still feed your gut bacteria but minimize fermentation side effects or IBS flare-ups.

Prebiotic Foods List

Fruit

- Apples
- Avocado
- Bananas
- Berries
- Cherries
- Green banana flour
- Kiwi
- Mango

Vegetables

- Asparagus

- Broccoli
- Cauliflower
- Dandelion greens
- Jerusalem artichokes / "sunchokes"
- Jicama root
- Konjac root
- Leeks
- Mushrooms
- Onions
- Peas
- Sweet potatoes
- Tomatoes
- Yacon root

Grains and Starches

- Amaranth
- Barley
- Buckwheat
- Cassava flour
- Oats
- Potatoes
- Quinoa
- Sweet potatoes
- Tapioca starch
- Wheat bran
- Whole wheat

Nuts and Seeds

- Almonds
- Chia seeds
- Flaxseeds
- Walnuts

Beans and legumes

- Black beans
- Chickpeas
- Lentils
- Pinto beans
- Peas
- Soybeans

Herbs and spices

- Burdock root
- Cacao powder
- Chicory root
- Dandelion root
- Garlic
- Green tea
- Licorice root
- Marshmallow root
- Psyllium husks
- Seaweed
- Slippery elm

- Triphala

Low-FODMAP Prebiotics

If you suffer from IBS or other intestinal discomfort when eating high-FODMAP foods, pick these low-FODMAP items instead:

- Almonds
- Berries
- Broccoli (if less than 1/2 cup per serving)
- Burdock root
- Cacao powder
- Cassava flour
- Chickpeas (if 1/4 cup cooked or less)
- Chia seeds
- Dandelion greens
- Flax meal (ground flax seeds)
- Ginger
- Green tea & matcha
- Kiwi
- Leeks
- Less than 1/2 cup of lentils
- Licorice root
- Peas
- Potatoes
- Psyllium husk powder
- Seaweed
- Sweet potatoes
- Tapioca starch

- Tomatoes
- Walnuts

Low-Fiber Prebiotics

Getting enough fiber is crucial for a healthy gut, but not everyone can handle a high-fiber diet. If you are sensitive to high-fiber foods or have gastrointestinal issues that are aggravated by fiber, opt for these low-fiber prebiotics:

- Almond butter
- Burdock root tea
- Cassava
- Cooked, skinless, seedless veggies
- Dandelion greens (cooked or juiced)
- Ginger root (juiced or extracted)
- Green peas (cooked)
- Green tea/matcha
- Licorice root
- Marshmallow root
- Potatoes (cooked and peeled)
- Raw honey
- Sweet potatoes (cooked and peeled)
- Tapioca
- Walnut butter
- Tomato paste (pureed)

Probiotics

Probiotics might sound similar to prebiotics, but they're very different. Probiotics are helpful bacteria and yeasts that may improve your gut health, and they're sometimes recommended to help with digestive issues, especially when taking antibiotic medications. Probiotics can be found in various food items and supplements, and there are three major types to be aware of:

- Lactobacillus: Found in fermented foods and yogurt, this is the most common probiotic and may help relieve symptoms of diarrhea and lactose intolerance.
- Saccharomyces boulardii: A probiotic yeast that may help alleviate symptoms of diarrhea and other digestive difficulties.
- Bifidobacterium: A probiotic that may help relieve symptoms of IBS and other digestive issues and is found in a few dairy products.

Probiotic Foods List

- Apple cider vinegar
- Apples
- Balsamic vinegar
- Bananas
- Beer
- Bottled probiotic drinks

- Celery juice
- Cereal
- Cheddar cheese
- Cottage cheese
- Dairy alternatives
- Dark chocolate
- Fermented fish
- Feta
- Garlic
- Gouda
- Greek yogurt
- Green peas
- Herbal teas
- Kefir
- Kimchi
- Kombucha
- Kvass
- Lassi
- Microalgae
- Miso
- Mozzarella
- Natto
- Olives
- Onions
- Parmesan
- Pickled beets
- Pickled cucumbers
- Pickled onions

- Provolone
- Raw cheeses
- Sauerkraut
- Skyr
- Smoothies
- Sour cream
- Sourdough bread
- Soy milk
- Soy sauce
- Spirulina
- Supplements
- Tempeh
- Traditional buttermilk
- Turshi
- Umeboshi
- Yogurt

Important note: Yogurt and Greek yogurt aren't quite the same. Yogurt is created when milk is fermented using bifidobacteria and lactic acid bacteria. Greek yogurt takes the process further and is a result of straining regular yogurt to increase the protein content and reduce the carbs and sugar.

Top tip: When shopping for foods containing probiotics, read the label and look for products that state they contain "live and active cultures".

FOODS THAT CAN HARM GUT HEALTH

A gut health-friendly diet isn't a strict or excessively restrictive diet. The focus should be on including or increasing your consumption of foods that promote gut health while decreasing or limiting foods that may be bad for your gut. You don't have to completely cut out any of the following foods (discussed in the following section), but you should scale back how much you include in your diet.

Processed Foods

Processed foods refer to any edible items that have been changed from their natural state in any way. This means that even cooking or drying food can be considered processing. However, what is usually meant when discussing unhealthy processed food is that it's been processed so much that it contains a load of additives, preservatives, fat, sugar, salt, and other ingredients. These foods are usually referred to as highly- or ultra-processed. Even foods that don't seem unhealthy may have been packed with added ingredients, such as tinned, bottled, and packaged goods. Here are some types of processed food and the reasons why they are potentially harmful to your gut:

Excess Sugar

Processed foods often contain added sugar, and including too many of these items can create a high-sugar diet even if you're not consuming lots of actual table sugar. Research into typical Western eating habits is ongoing, and emerging evidence links diets rich in refined sugars with gut dysbiosis and metabolic diseases. Consuming lots of sugar can damage the gastrointestinal lining and lower levels of crucial immune cells. It can also tip the balance in favor of non-beneficial bacteria that instigate inflammation throughout the body by decreasing the populations of beneficial bacteria that support healthy immune function (Berman, 2022).

Artificial Sweeteners

Since consuming too much sugar can be bad for your overall health, you may think that swapping to sugar-free options that contain artificial sweeteners is the way to go. Unfortunately, that's not the case, as artificial sweeteners aren't really any healthier than sugar. Research into the effects of the increasing use of artificial sweeteners on consumers is ongoing, but evidence is emerging that they are not conducive to health. Studies are finding that higher intake of various artificial sweeteners can disrupt the gut microbiome, making it harder for beneficial bacteria to survive. These sweeteners are also linked to an increase in non-beneficial microbe populations, which may increase the risk of gastrointestinal problems and metabolic disease (Shil & Chichger, 2021).

Dietary Emulsifiers

Emulsifiers are substances added to processed foods that help to combine two ingredients that would naturally separate. If you've ever tried to mix oil and water together, you'll know it won't happen naturally, but if you add an emulsifier, they'll mix and stay mixed. They're common in a variety of processed foods, including ice cream, mayonnaise, and margarine. While this may offer opportunities to create delicious packaged foods that remain perfectly combined, it doesn't do your gut any good. Research suggests that emulsifiers may harm the mucous lining that separates gut bacteria from the walls of the gastrointestinal tract. Damage to this mucous lining not only causes inflammation but may allow bacteria that should stay in the gut to escape and cause inflammation elsewhere in the body, which increases the risk of inflammatory disease (Chassaing et al., 2015).

Excess Sodium

Salt and sodium are often confused as being one and the same, possibly because the chemical name for salt is sodium chloride. Sodium is not salt but an element and is a component of the mineral found in table salt. Like sugar, salt is used to flavor processed foods and can be found in a wide range of products, from baked goods to cured meats to canned food. The problem with sodium is that an excessive intake has been linked to tissue inflammation in the gut and rest of the body and disruption of the gut microbiome, which may increase the risk of various inflammatory diseases, including hypertension and heart disease (Smiljanec & Lennon, 2018).

Soy

Soy has been farmed and eaten by humans for thousands of years and has many applications in the food production industry. From being used as a meat or dairy substitute to having emulsifying properties, soy is found in a variety of processed foods. Unfortunately, despite being a plant-based ingredient, it often has to undergo a lot of processing. These high levels of processing have altered how the ingredient interacts with the body. It's been found that soy-based foods have the potential to negatively impact the gut microbiome and microbe populations. Often, overall bacteria numbers aren't greatly affected, but individual populations are, showing significant decreases or increases that may contribute to gut function issues (Gill & Uno, 2016).

Unfermented Dairy

Unfermented dairy or dairy derivatives include products such as milk, whey protein, and ice cream. Fermented dairy products include yogurt, sour cream, and cultured butter-milk. The fermentation process creates different dairy foods from a single source. It helps extend a product's shelf life to avoid waste and makes the food better for your gut. Unfermented dairy, however, can be bad for your gut health by causing disruptions to the microbe populations and their environment. Some proteins found in unfermented dairy or dairy derivatives can cause inflammation in the gut and gastrointestinal issues that may decrease the number of beneficial bacteria and boost populations of detrimental bacteria.

Red Meat

Humans are omnivores, so including animal products, such as meat, in our diet is natural. However, animal proteins aren't all the same, and some kinds are potentially harmful to your gut health if consumed in large amounts or consumed too often; red meat is one of them. Studies have indicated that eating large amounts of red meat, or eating it too often can disrupt the balance between gut bacterial species. A red meat-rich diet has been shown to lower the number of beneficial bacteria while simultaneously creating an environment that increases the number of potentially harmful bacteria that may cause inflammation by damaging the lining of the gastrointestinal tract (Murphey, Velazquez & Herbert, 2015).

Alcohol

Consuming too much alcohol is associated with a variety of health risks, from hypertension to liver disease, but it can also affect your gut health. Research has shown the harmful effects of excessive or frequent alcohol consumption on gut bacteria, the intestinal lining, and gut inflammation. It's also been suggested that the adverse effects can be lessened by quitting or scaling back on alcohol consumption (Ames et al., 2018).

MEAL PLANNING

Understanding what a gut-healthy diet should be, and understanding which foods go the extra mile to support your gut, and which foods can be harmful, are the first steps to take to clean up your eating habits for the better.

However, this knowledge alone isn't enough to help you implement and stick to the necessary dietary changes. You need a plan that you can follow to make your life easier and help you maintain healthy changes. Meal planning is the solution.

Meal planning is critical to a healthy lifestyle and good time management. If you've never tried meal planning or are skeptical about whether it's really worth it, here's what science has to say about the efficacy and benefits of planning your meals in advance.

Meal planning may improve the quality and variety of foods you eat. People who prepare home-cooked meals using nutritious ingredients are more likely to eat higher-quality meals and a wider variety than those who rely on ready meals, takeout, or whatever they happen to have on hand at mealtimes (Ducrot et al., 2017). Part of the reason for this is that pre-planning meals usually encourages individuals to get more creative and include different ingredients instead of falling back on the same recipes or ingredients they're used to preparing or keeping in their kitchen. Preparing meals daily is also associated with consuming healthier, plant-based ingredients or meals, such as fruit, vegetables, and salads (Monsivais, Aggarwal & Drewnowski, 2014). Further research has identified that pre-planning meals for the week ahead encourage people to stick to healthy eating habits and make better, more nutritious food choices than if they were making meal decisions impulsively (Fruh, 2013).

Planning your meals doesn't just help you stick to your gut-healthy eating habits. It can also help you shed a few pounds and keep them off, which, in turn, benefits your gut health. You'll likely cut excess calories, sodium, sugar, and fat from your diet by swapping takeout, ready meals, and processed foods for fresh ingredients. This, in combination with portion control and regular physical activity, sets you up to prevent unwanted weight gain or trim down to a healthier body fat percentage. Science is amassing more and more evidence that suggests obesity and gut dysbiosis are linked. Individuals who carry more body fat tend to have less diverse gut bacteria and fewer beneficial microbe species than their leaner counterparts (Pinart et al., 2021). Conversely, an unbalanced gut could contribute to obesity by skewing microbe populations in favor of bacteria that encourage weight gain. When the populations of these microbes outweigh the populations of other beneficial bacteria, they're likely to increase the appetite, and in the amount of energy absorbed from food, and also increase the storage of that additional energy as fat (Liu et al., 2021).

Finally, meal planning and prepping have even been associated with having mental and emotional benefits. Studies have found a positive correlation between spending time preparing meals daily and an increased sense of mental wellness while lowering feelings of stress (Widener et al., 2021). It's also suggested that planning meals ahead of time takes the weight of in-the-moment decision-making off a person's shoulders, reducing feelings of anxiety, which also lowers blood pressure (Osdoba et al., 2014).

With so many great reasons to start pre-planning your meals, there's no good excuse to put off getting into this positive habit. You could start today!

How To Meal Plan

Before rushing to take the steps of effective meal planning, it's important to debunk some misconceptions and define what meal planning is (but first it's important to say what meal planning isn't). Misconceptions often act as mental obstacles to adopting meal planning as a healthy lifestyle habit.

Meal planning isn't:

- Having a giant week-by-week binder of the entire month's meals planned in advance
- Expensive compared to impulse food choices
- Only valid for families with several mouths to feed
- Eating home-cooked meals all the time
- Inflexible; it is not imperative that you can only eat what you planned to eat for any given meal on a particular day
- Too much work for busy people

Meal planning is:

- taking the guesswork out of "What's for dinner/lunch/breakfast?" for a week in advance
- Shopping weekly for ingredients instead of wasting time in the grocery aisles every day

- Preparing ingredients in advance to make cooking quick and easy

Steps to Effective Meal Planning

Meal planning can be done in a few easy steps that don't have to take up too much of your time, or deplete your mental bandwidth, or become complicated. Before starting the actual meal planning, decide why you want to do it. Consider the following questions:

- Do you want more dietary variety?
- Do you want to stick to healthier eating goals?
- Do you want to cut costs and eat well on a budget?
- Do you want to improve your time management, especially on busy weeknights?
- Do you want to take the hassle and anxiety out of deciding to eat every single meal every day?

Whether you have one or several reasons for wanting to start meal planning, understanding why you're putting in the effort will motivate you to do it.

Decide how many meals: Pick the meals you want to plan for. Perhaps you only want to pre-plan one meal per day or maybe two or all three.

Decide what you need from individual meals: Think about your week's schedule. If you're going to get home late one night, you might want to make a slow-cooked meal that day so it's ready and waiting when you get home. You might want to take leftovers to work for lunch on days you're too busy to prepare lunch the night before or the morning of. Decide what you need from each meal you're planning for.

Choose your recipes: Choose recipes that will work for you, such as picking recipes that make enough to have leftovers, can be done in the slow cooker while you're at work, or can be thrown together in a flash. Choose recipes you know you enjoy, and choose at least one new one per week. To make your life easier, choose recipes that share common staple ingredients to cut down on wastage. Just be sure to switch up your staple ingredients from week to week to maintain variety in your diet.

Make smart grocery lists: Start by listing all the ingredients you'll need for the week's meal, and then go through your kitchen to cross off any ingredients you already have and don't need more of.

Prepare ingredients ahead of time: Set aside an hour the day before your work week starts. Use this hour to pre-chop and pre-cook ingredients in batches to store in the fridge. It'll reduce meal prep time on the day of making the meal.

Meal Planning Tips for One

Meal planning and cooking for a single person is an incon-venience and is often a deterrent for people living on their own to make home-cooked meals. The good news is that eating well and meal planning for one doesn't have to be a headache when you follow these tips:

- Pick recipes that are meant to serve only one or two people. There will be less wastage, and recipes for two will give you leftovers to reheat another day.
- Portion out and freeze meat immediately. It's not always possible to buy meat in single portion sizes, but you can cut it up into portions, freeze it, and defrost only what you need when you need it.
- Shop for ingredients at the salad bar. Often canned, pre-packed, or even whole fresh vegetables and other ingredients can be more than you actually need. By shopping at the store's salad bar, you can measure precisely the amount you need and avoid wastage.
- Freeze leftovers from large meals immediately. Cranking up the oven for one or two portions of baked meals can seem like a huge waste of time and electricity. If you make a casserole, lasagna, or any other meal that makes a large amount, take out two portions and freeze the rest. You don't have to eat the same thing every night for a whole week, you get to enjoy recipes that don't specifically serve one or two, and you'll have food that can just be reheated if you run out of time on a hectic day.
- Roast a large batch of vegetables at once. You don't have to spend ages prepping and roasting vegetables daily or even every other day. Roast a big batch at once, portion them out, and have them ready to reheat when you need them as sides during the week.

- Make meals that offer leftovers. Leftovers can be stowed away in the fridge for another night or taken to work the next day for lunch.
- Use staple ingredients that can be repurposed for several meals. For example, roasted or grilled chicken can be prepped ahead of time and portioned up for different meals throughout the week. The chicken could be used in dishes such as salads, tacos, sandwiches, and more. Using the same base ingredients in many ways will save cooking time and prevent wastage.

Grocery Shopping Tips

Grocery shopping is an integral part of meal planning. Use these tips to avoid common shopping pitfalls to shop smarter and make meal planning easier:

Don't shop hungry: Hunger can play tricks on your brain by making your thoughts less clear. This can lead to buying unnecessary items based on hunger and cravings.

Check for sales online: You can get a heads up about what's on sale and reduce the time spent checking for any sales on items you need while browsing the aisles. You might also decide to visit a different store because they stock items that you want that are cheaper than your usual store, or have been reduced in price.

Organize your shopping list by aisle or department: There's nothing more annoying than having to scan through your entire list in each aisle or traipse back and forth to aisles you've already been in because there's something further down the list you needed from there.

Consider frozen foods: Frozen foods often come in blended packets or containers that offer a mix of veggies or grains you can pop on the stove or in the microwave, saving preparation time and increasing variety.

Consider canned foods: Canned items may not be as good as the fresh foods, but they could be useful if you are short of time. Having canned ingredients for some meals can save time and improve meal preparation efficiency.

Splurge on convenience: Convenience items, such as salad kits or packages of peeled diced fruit or vegetables may cost more, but the expense may be offset by the benefits. They save you time making your meal, and, in some cases, they come in single-serving portions to cut back on wastage if you're cooking for one, or if you only need a small amount.

WHAT'S NEXT?

Fueling your body with the correct nutrition is vital for physical and mental wellness. No single diet is the "one true way" to achieve optimal health, but some diets are generally better than others. It is up to you personally to create a diet that provides all the nutrition you need and makes you feel good. You should be aiming for a balanced diet that incorporates probiotics, prebiotics, and gut-healthy supplements while minimizing potentially harmful foods.

That being said, there is no reason to completely eliminate any foods from your diet altogether, or try to force yourself to adapt to any popular extreme diet just because there are enthusiasts who champion such plans. Your diet must be easy to follow, and filled with foods that support gut and mental health that you like. If there are certain healthy foods you can't stand, that's okay. Don't try to include them in your diet. If there are some potentially unhealthy foods that you absolutely love, that's also fine. Don't try to completely eliminate them from your life, as you'll only end up feeling deprived and unhappy, which isn't good for your physical or mental wellness. The focus should be on what you eat and how much you eat. Opt for eating more foods that support health and minimizing those that may impede wellness so that you create a diet you are comfortable with, and that you will be able to stick to.

Once you've identified foods you want to eat more of, and ingredients you want to start including, and things you want to cut back on, you can try meal planning. Changing your diet isn't easy. Diet is like a habit; different foods have ingredients that make them more appealing to consumers, reinforcing poor dietary choices. Stress and a busy lifestyle can make breaking old eating habits and replacing them with new, healthier ones even more difficult. Planning may be your "meal ticket" to easily and effectively making dietary changes that last.

Nutrition isn't alone in the war on an unhealthy gut and mind. It's one piece of the jigsaw puzzle that creates a bigger picture of holistic health. The next chapter will focus on physically supporting gut health and mental wellness. This refers to the physical things you can do, specifically exercise and sleep. These factors are enormous contributors; you'll discover why and how they impact your wellbeing. We'll also cover some types of exercise that are particularly beneficial and tips for increasing physical activity and for improving your sleep habits to boost gut wellness and mental health.

CHANGING THE WORLD ONE GUT
AND MIND AT A TIME

The gut-brain axis, or more specifically, the microbe-gut-brain axis, is a naturally occurring human physiological communication highway that we have been aware of for centuries. Despite this, it's only recently come to prominence under the investigation of modern medicine and medicinal science. The more technology advances, the more we learn about the human body and how it works. What we previously had an awareness of is now proven and elaborated on, and this knowledge continues to be built up as more research is done and further intricacies of our physiological inner workings are discovered. However, just because researchers and scientists make these discoveries doesn't mean everyone is learning about them. For many, the gut-brain axis is still an utterly enigmatic mystery. Sure, you may inherently know that your mind and gut are connected because you've experienced those nervous butterflies or stress-related digestive upset. That's just a vague awareness of the link, though.

You are beginning to understand how connected your gut and mind are. You're learning of the power of the gut-brain axis and its effect on your entire wellbeing if either part of the axis is not as healthy as it should be. This understanding still escapes many people, and without that crucial knowledge, others can never achieve optimal health. Only when knowledge, understanding, and a clear vision of the needed changes come together can someone alter their lifestyle to transform their health and their experience of life.

Health, wellbeing, and a positive experience of life are invaluable. Since knowledge is the path to these things, knowledge itself is priceless. In modern times, society emphasizes the guarding of what we have, and keeping them to ourselves, in a bid to preserve power and have the "upper hand". Society doesn't seem to recognize that some things are meant to be shared and are beneficial to share. Knowledge is one of them.

By sharing the knowledge you are gaining, you are not losing a valuable commodity but rather facilitating an increased sense of wellbeing and enjoyment of life. When you help those around you, and even those you may never meet, you are playing a role in creating a healthier, happier, and, therefore, better world and society. Others play a significant role in how we personally experience life and can even impact our personal health and wellbeing, as you'll discover later in this guide.

Positive change in our own lives and the world at large starts with individuals making positive changes; it is the pebble and ripple effect. Sharing the knowledge you are gaining is like throwing a pebble into water, and positive change is like the ripples from that pebble. If you want to be part of changing the world for the better, one person, one gut, and one mind at a time, feel free to throw that pebble into the water by sharing your experience of the knowledge you are gaining. **By leaving a review, you will help alert others to the value of this book and help spread awareness and encourage others to make similar positive changes in their lives, which could ultimately affect those around them and even you.**

Please visit the link below or scan the QR code to leave feedback on Amazon.

https://www.amazon.com/review/create-review/?asin=1738431223

4

PART 3: PHYSICALLY SUPPORTING GUT HEALTH AND MENTAL WELLNESS

Healthy lifestyle habits bolster physical and mental health and play a role in the prevention of chronic health issues. This chapter will focus on healthy lifestyle changes that improve and support physical, mental, and gut health. These lifestyle changes primarily deal with the physical approach to wellbeing. In the next chapter, we'll focus on approaches that deal more with the mental and emotional aspects.

The positive lifestyle habits that support mental health and wellbeing, which we will be tackling in this chapter, are:

- Physical activity or exercise
- Healthy sleep habits

EXERCISE AND GUT HEALTH

Exercise is a large part of a healthy lifestyle for both physical and mental wellness. Some benefits of regular exercise are pretty well known, while others don't get as much attention. For example, you've probably been told about the benefits for your major muscle groups, cardiovascular system, and other things like blood pressure and weight maintenance. What you may not know is that exercise is also beneficial for your gut in various ways, including:

Regulating bowel movements: It's not just your prominent and visible muscles that get a workout when you exercise. The muscles lining your gastrointestinal tract are also strengthened, improving the contractions to keep things moving smoothly from one end to the other.

Improving immune function: Regular exercise enhances and regulates your immune response and is an anti-inflammatory mechanism to reduce or prevent chronic systemic inflammation. Research backs up these claims by highlighting the relationship between moderate-intensity exercise and a reduced risk of illness (Nieman & Wentz, 2019).

Reducing stress: We've discussed the impact of stress on gut health, and exercise can help you reduce and manage your stress levels. It does this in two steps. The amount of stress hormones in your body, including cortisol and adrenaline, are lowered. Endorphins, nature's feel-good chemical, are released during exercise, acting as a natural painkiller and mood booster.

Improving the gut microbiome: Besides influencing gut health, research suggests that exercise may even directly improve your gut bacteria by increasing the number of beneficial species (Monda et al., 2017).

EXERCISE AND MENTAL WELLNESS

Exercise can be as good for your mind as it is for your body. It improves your mental wellness, cognition, and the physical health of your brain. Studies have linked regular physical activity to lowering anxiety, improving mood, and alleviating symptoms of depression. It's also been shown to boost self-esteem and reduce the social withdrawal associated with poor self-esteem (Sharma, Madaan & Petty, 2006).

When it comes to physical activity, there is no one true "best" exercise specifically for gut health. Your gut will benefit from any form of activity as long as you get your body moving and muscles working. However, two types of exercise are great for overall health and wellbeing are aerobic exercise and yoga. They can range from easy to complex.

AEROBIC ACTIVITY

Aerobic activity is any physical activity that gets your heart rate and breathing up. When people hear the term "aerobic exercise," they typically think of running or of aerobics classes. However, it can be anything that works your respiratory and cardiovascular system, even walking. Yes, walking is overlooked and underestimated as an effective form of exercise. One of the great things about walking is that it's suitable for a wide variety of people across all age groups, fitness levels, and physical capabilities, thanks to its low-impact nature. In fact, if you want to know more about how walking can transform your life by improving your health, fitness, and aiding weight loss, check out *Walking Your Way to Weight Loss: A Simple Two-Part Approach to Becoming Fitter, Healthier, and Happier in 49 Days*, which is available through Amazon! The book details the extensive benefits of walking and guides readers through the various types of walking. It is a beginner's guide to get them started on their journey to improving health and wellbeing by simply putting one foot in front of the other!

Aerobic activity isn't just good for your cardiovascular and respiratory health. It's also good for your mental wellness. Science suggests that out of different types of physical activity, aerobic exercise shows the most substantial impact on treating and alleviating symptoms of depression (Myers, 2023).

YOGA

Most people are at least vaguely familiar with yoga. They may draw the mental image of someone contorting their bodies into seemingly impossible positions like a human pretzel. While this mainstream idea can sometimes be the reality, the truth is far from it. Yoga is a form of physical and mental exercise that utilizes various poses, controlled breathing, and a meditative influence to provide a holistic workout for body, mind, and spirit. Contrary to the popular image of advanced poses, yoga is for everyone, irrespective of age, weight, flexibility, or fitness. The poses range from simple to advanced, allowing anyone to progress from beginner to pro over time.

The physical aspect of yoga effectively improves coordination, muscle strength, flexibility, and balance, but that's not all. The mental side of the practice is associated with stress relief and management. Yoga can help you lower the amount of stress hormones in your body while boosting the levels of beneficial chemicals in your brain that help improve your mood, reduce anxiety, and relieve depression (Muck, 2021).

The trick with yoga is to find a style that suits your needs, starting with the easiest poses, then work your way up to more challenging ones. There are dozens of different styles of yoga, with some being more popular or suitable than others. Take your time to find which style is best for you, but in the meantime, get started with these beginner-friendly poses to start strengthening your mind and body today.

Important note: Whenever practicing yoga, only perform the pose as far as is comfortable for you. Don't try to force your body into a position that isn't comfortable, as this could lead to injury, the complete opposite of what you're trying to achieve.

Child's Pose

- Assume a kneeling position on the ground with your knees together.
- Sit back on your heels while reaching your arms above your head.
- Bend forward from the hips, lowering your forehead to the ground while extending your arms, palms facing down, keeping your bottom resting on your calves and heels.

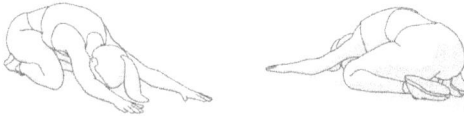

Why do it: To gently stretch your spine, neck, hips, and shoulders.

When to skip it: If you are pregnant, hypertensive, or have knee or ankle issues.

How to modify it: Put a rolled towel under your ankles and rest your head on a cushion or yoga block to make the stretch less deep.

What to focus on: Relaxing the muscles along your back.

Plank Pose

- Kneel on the ground on all fours with your knees together.
- Lean forward until your shoulders are over your wrists.
- Extend one leg backward with your toes tucked, shifting your weight onto that leg, and then extend the other leg backward.
- Keep your body in a straight diagonal line from shoulders to ankles – you should be in a high push-up position.

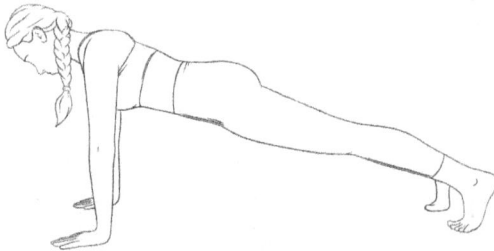

Why do it: To increase core, shoulder, arm, and leg strength.

When to skip it: If you suffer from carpal tunnel syndrome or have lower back pain.

How to modify it: Hold the pose on all fours and lean forward to align your shoulders and wrists without extending your legs backward.

What to focus on: Imagining your spine lengthening as you breathe into the pose.

Tree Pose

- Stand with your feet together and your hands together in front of your chest, palms facing each other.
- Bend your right knee, raising your knee out sideways to bring the sole of your right foot up to your inner left thigh above the knee.
- Lower your right foot back to the ground, toes facing forward, and repeat the previous step on the left side.

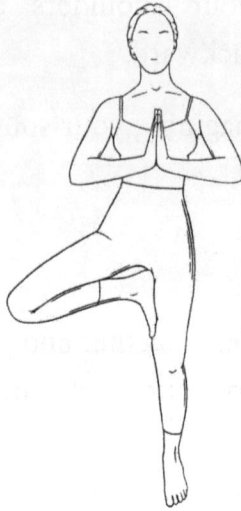

Why do it: To improve balance, strength, and posture.

When to skip it: If you suffer from hypotension or medical conditions causing balance problems.

How to modify it: Perform the pose, bear a wall, chair, or counter, and place your hands on the sturdy surface for support while developing your balance.

What to focus on: Breathing evenly.

Cobra Pose

- Lie flat on your stomach on the ground, legs together.

- Bend your elbows and place your hands, palms down, in line with your shoulders, and as close to your body as possible.
- Push up through your palms and tighten the upper back muscles, raising your chest off the floor while looking straight ahead and maintaining a neutral head and neck position.

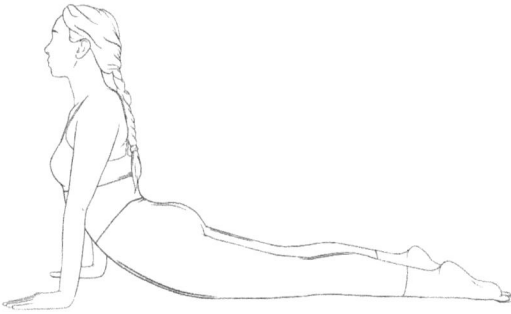

Why do it: To increase back strength.

When to skip it: If you suffer from carpal tunnel syndrome, shoulder or wrist issues, or back pain.

How to modify it: Raise your chest off the ground only as far as comfortable. You don't have to fully straighten your arms.

What to focus on: Pressing your pelvis into the ground and drawing your navel upwards away from the ground as you raise your chest up.

Bridge Pose

- Lie on your back on the ground with your feet hip-width apart and your arms extended alongside your body, palms facing down.
- Bend your knees to bring your feet as close to your bottom as possible.
- Draw your hips and navel up to form a straight diagonal line between your knees and shoulders while keeping your feet flat on the ground.
- Tuck your chin toward your chest slightly and bring your hands together beneath you, interlacing your fingers.

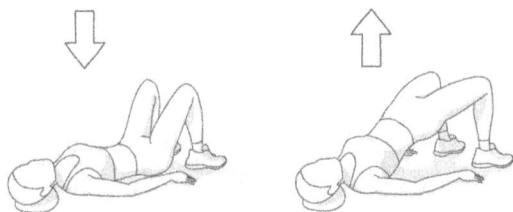

Why do it: To open your upper chest to relieve tension caused by sitting for long periods.

When to skip it: If you have a neck injury.

How to modify it: Place a yoga block between your thighs to maintain correct alignment of your hips, knees, and feet.

What to focus on: Raising your chest away from the ground if you can, using your shoulder blades as the contact point with the ground.

TIPS FOR ADDING PHYSICAL ACTIVITY TO YOUR LIFESTYLE

If you're not particularly active, improving your fitness can be a real challenge. Finding it difficult to add physical activity to your lifestyle doesn't mean you're lazy. Let's face it: it can be challenging and uncomfortable when you're just starting out, which doesn't do much to bolster your resolve and motivation. You need to make it as easy for yourself to get active and stay active. So, here are some tips for incorporating exercise into your lifestyle:

Plan ahead: Decide what to do and when to do it. Mark it in your daily planner so you're more likely to schedule things around it, lay out your workout clothes, download your podcast or playlist, for example, and plan a snack or meal to eat before or after your workout.

Make it convenient: The less fuss involved, such as setting up lots of equipment or driving miles to a class, the better. The more convenient the exercise is, the fewer excuses you'll find to skip it.

Start small: Some activity is better than no activity. You can't go from couch potato to athlete overnight. Yogis didn't learn fancy poses until they had mastered the easier ones. Set smaller goals that lead to larger ones.

Enjoy it: Pick activities and yoga poses you like or that offer specific benefits you want.

Keep track of progress: Measuring your progress is a huge motivator to keep at it or to set bigger goals to keep improving.

Get social: Find a workout class, a yoga group,, or a workout buddy to keep you company and make things more enjoyable.

SLEEP AND GUT HEALTH

Sleep isn't just crucial for keeping crankiness at bay. It's vital for various health reasons, not least your gut health. Not getting sufficient quality sleep can affect your gut in several ways.

Stress: Not getting enough sleep can increase stress and lead to hormonal imbalance and a rise in cortisol levels.

Diet: Sleep deprivation can upset your hunger hormones, leading to increased appetite. Combine that with tiredness-induced poor decision-making, and you could find yourself reaching for unhealthy foods as a quick energy source.

GERD: Gastroesophageal reflux disease is when stomach acid repeatedly flows out of the stomach and up the esophagus or the lower part of the throat that leads to the stomach. This is usually referred to as acid reflux. Lack of sleep can decrease how much melatonin is produced in your body, and this drop in the hormone can lead to developing GERD.

Continued research is beginning to link sleep quality with a healthy gut microbiome and vice versa. A study published in The European Journal of Nutrition suggests that irregular or poor sleeping habits are associated with increased harmful gut bacteria populations (Bermingham et al., 2023). Conversely, other research has shown a link between a healthy gut and improved sleep quality (Smith et al., 2019).

SLEEP AND MENTAL WELLNESS

Getting a good night's sleep supports your physical health, mental health, and cognition. Being sleep-deprived may actually alter some brain activity, making it harder to think and regulate your emotions. Changes in these brain activities are associated with:

- Decision-making difficulties
- Lack of mental clarity
- Poor problem solving
- Impulse and behavior control issues
- Difficulty regulating emotions and emotional responses
- Poor adaptation to change
- Depression
- Increased risk-taking behavior
- Suicidal ideations

(How Sleep Affects Your Health, 2022)

TIPS FOR GETTING BETTER SLEEP

As you can see, sleep is a vital part of overall health and well-being. However, our modern world doesn't do much to encourage healthy sleeping habits. It is difficult to get enough sleep of good quality. Here's how to improve your sleep habits and the quality of your sleep.

Be consistent: The human body is hardwired to prefer consistent regular routines. To take advantage of this physiological and mental preference, maintain a regular sleep schedule so your body develops the intuition to start winding down for bedtime at a usual time, sleep regular hours, and wake up at a standard time.

Sleep enough hours: Every vertebrate on the planet needs a certain amount of sleep for optimal health. It can be anywhere from 7-9 hours for humans, with exceptions on either side of that average. Make sure you schedule at least 7 hours of sleep per night, more if you personally need it to feel your best. It's vital to note that sleep hours mean quality sleep, not broken sleep.

Observe circadian rhythms: A circadian rhythm is a natural 24-hour physiological cycle in most creatures. It's also referred to as your body's internal clock, and it's a natural response to the wake-sleep cycle prompted by the time of day. Many creatures will wake up when their environment becomes light enough to see and carry out their business and will go to sleep when night falls, and they can no longer see. There are a few exceptions to the rules, such as nocturnal creatures (which are most active at night) or crepuscular creatures (which are most active during the twilight hours). However, humans are generally diurnal, meaning we are most active during daylight hours. This lends itself to a natural tendency to wake up in response to light and get sleepy in response to fading light.

Most importantly, it must be noted that you don't just climb into bed and go to sleep for the night. A process is usually involved, activated by the decreasing light and temperature around you, that signals your body to prepare for the sleep cycle. In our modern world, however, we have artificial light, blue light from electronic devices, and disruptions to our diurnal nature with obligations such as shift work. All of this opposes, and can derail, our circadian rhythms. To make it easier for your body to prepare for and accommodate quality sleep physiologically, try to align your sleep habits with your body's natural circadian rhythm.

Cut back on screen time: Between the artificial light we illuminate our homes with and the light-emitting devices we have become entirely dependent on, our natural circadian rhythms are completely out of alignment. Our eyes detect light, and that's part of what stimulates our bodily wakefulness. As creatures who are supposed to rise with the sun and head for bed at sunset, the presence of light plays a pivotal role in our wake-sleep cycles. Artificial light and, specifically, the type of light emitted from the electronic devices we use into the night hours, such as cell phones and television, interfere with our natural sleep patterns. Accommodate a natural, circadian rhythm sleep pattern by cutting back on screen time before bed. If possible, avoid screens when the sun starts setting and use dimmer lights to mimic natural fading light into the evening before bed.

Remove electronics from the bedroom: From screens that light up when you get notifications to the sounds accompanying them, many electronics have an incredible propensity to disturb your sleep. Leave electronics such as cell phones and tablets charging in another room overnight. Outlaw televisions and ban laptops from your bedroom. Your bedroom should be a sleep sanctuary, making the light and noise disturbances during your sleep hours "illegal". Additionally, just the fact that the devices are in the room can cause anxiety and tempt you to check them for notifications and messages when you do wake up during the night, preventing you from falling back to sleep with ease. No electronics of any sort should be in the bedroom if you want to create a space that not only facilitates but encourages sleep.

Make your bedroom inviting: Aside from removing most electronics, it's vital to create a space that makes you feel safe, relaxed, and comfortable. Being physically and mentally comfortable and relaxed makes falling and staying asleep easier. It's about more than just your bed and pillows. Darkness, a comfortable temperature, and either silence or soothing sounds will aid in falling asleep and reduce sleep disturbances.

Get physical: Physical activity may help you get a better night's sleep. Exercise enables you to burn off energy and decrease the time you spend lying awake in bed staring at the ceiling while waiting to fall asleep. It also contributes to stress reduction and management, which can curb sleep disturbances caused by worry and anxiety. Even gentle or low-intensity physical activity can do the trick, but if you opt for high-intensity exercise, ensure it's several hours before bedtime.

Maintain a consistent routine: Routines provide cues for both body and mind about what to expect next. Consistency is vital and includes following the same or similar steps each night at roughly the same time. Try dimming the lights, winding down with restful activities like listening to pleasant music or reading, and getting physically comfortable.

Get back to sleep easier: If you find yourself waking up in the middle of the night and you're having trouble getting back to sleep, try these tips to fall back asleep more easily:

- Don't look at the time. Watching the minutes tick by may cause worry and anxiety over getting enough sleep, which can actually wake your brain up, keeping you awake for longer.
- Try meditation or a relaxation exercise. Calming your body and mind may cue you to continue sleeping peacefully.
- Use visualizations as a distraction. When you can't sleep, you might obsess over your inability to do so, or your mind might drift to stressful thoughts,

increasing your anxiety. Use relaxing visualizations to distract your mind from worry or anxiety and encourage it to focus on calm and rest.

- Listen to something. Whether soothing sounds, calming music, or even guided meditation, focusing on something soft to listen to helps distract and calm your mind.
- Get out of bed. If you're not having any luck falling back to sleep after 15-20 minutes, the frustration could cause your brain to associate your bedroom, which is your sleep sanctuary, with poor sleep. Try getting up and moving to another room to read, meditate, listen to music, or do other relaxing activities until you feel ready to go back to bed.

Things to avoid: There are numerous ways to improve your sleep habits and quality, but there are also some things you should not do, such as:

- Napping: As tempting as forty winks may seem when you're tired during the day, it can be detrimental to a healthy sleep schedule. Naps could make it harder to fall asleep and stay asleep during the night.
- Consuming caffeine and alcohol: Caffeine and alcohol are stimulants. Caffeine has a reputation for its energizing effect. Alcohol, on the other hand, may be associated with having a relaxing effect. However, the initial relaxation doesn't last, and it could end up

increasing anxiety and contributing to sleep disturbances. Limit or avoid alcohol and caffeine for several hours before bed.

- Eating heavy meals: Consuming a large meal can make you feel lazy and sleepy because all your body's energy is directed toward digestion. Digestion, however, can interrupt your sleep. After all, instead of relaxing and resting, your body is hard at work trying to process what you ate. Eat dinner a few hours before bed, and if you are really hungry, keep snacks small and light if you are eating close to bedtime.
- Drinking lots of fluids: Getting enough fluids during the day is healthy for your body, but downing several glasses of water shortly before bed can leave you sleepless. Drinking too much fluid before bed could see you waking up several times during the night to go to the bathroom, breaking crucial sleep cycles.

WHAT'S NEXT

In a world that has become dominated by convenience, technology, and an increasing number of sedentary jobs, it's no wonder that people tend to sit more and move less these days. All this time spent in a seat is taking its toll. Physical activity is crucial for health and wellbeing. Much of the time, the focus on the benefits of exercise is placed on how it's good for your body. It can reduce the risk of lifestyle-related health problems such as hypertension and cardiovascular disease. Its positive effects on your gut and mental wellness are not often among the top listed reasons to get more active.

However, considering the incredible role the gut-brain axis plays in someone's overall physical and mental wellbeing, they should be. Physical activity offers a crucial positive influence on your digestive system and your mind. The best part is that you don't have to spend hours sweating it out on a treadmill or push yourself to physical extremes with intimidating intense workout routines. Even simple and gentle activities, such as yoga and walking, can exert a positive impact. Suppose you're not a fan of running, your knees protest, you're physically uncomfortable doing it, and your mind questions your sanity when you do try running. In that case, it's really only an exercise in futility. The point is to get moving at an intensity you are comfortable with and doing activities you enjoy. Comfort + enjoyment = developing physical activity habits that are maintainable long term.

In conjunction with regular exercise, sleep plays a monumental role in physical and mental wellness. To demonstrate the influence a lack of sleep can have, think back to the last time you got less sleep than usual or just had a poor night's sleep and how you felt the next day. You probably felt tired and cranky, had difficulty concentrating and thinking clearly, and maybe even felt unwell. That was just one night of inadequate sleep. Now, compound the problem by getting too little or poor quality sleep every night over a long period of time. Eventually, you're likely to chronically feel physically fatigued and mentally drained, which can increase your risk of making poor decisions about sticking to healthy lifestyle changes and even impact your mental and emotional state.

Aside from mindfulness, the first three parts of your journey toward improved gut health and mental wellness mainly looked at physical strategies. It's time to delve deeper into other mental and emotional practices to enhance mental wellness and improve gut health via the gut-brain axis. Mindfulness does bring a mental aspect into your journey, but it's a particular type of strategy that cannot tackle a broader range of ways in which to support health mentally and emotionally. Mindfulness techniques can boost mental and emotional strategies, but they won't be successful on their own. In the next part, we will complete the four pillars that support gut health and mental wellness by looking at how you can support your health mentally and emotionally. These approaches are just as vital as the physical ones we've mentioned because of the two-way communication and effect of the gut-brain axis. When one improves, it's a step toward improving the other and vice versa. A healthy mind goes a long way to maintaining a healthy body, and a healthy mind is easier to maintain when the body is healthy.

5

PART 4: MENTALLY AND EMOTIONALLY SUPPORTING GUT HEALTH AND MENTAL WELLNESS

If you take a moment to look around you at the promotion of health, you will likely find that much of what you see focuses on physical health. Increasingly, mental and emotional health are coming into the limelight, but not as much or as regularly, or as prominently as they should be. Your health comprises what you can see, your physical body, and what you can't see, your mental and emotional inner workings. As you've discovered, when it comes to the gut-brain axis and holistic wellbeing, you can follow a healthy lifestyle and have what appears to be a healthy body but could still suffer the physical effects of poor mental health. You must also invest in your mental and emotional wellness to attain true wellbeing.

There are many different ways to improve and maintain mental and emotional health. During this part of the guide, you will read about a couple of popular and effective approaches. These approaches don't just highlight what you, personally, can do to increase wellbeing, but also how your relationships affect you. After all, you could invest all your effort in looking after your mental wellness, but the effort will lose efficacy if you don't address your social and personal relationships. We're also going to zone in on the power of positivity and how to attract and cultivate more of it in your life, simultaneously combatting the negativity that is often associated with depression and anxiety.

THE PRINCIPLES OF POSITIVE PSYCHOLOGY

Positive psychology can have many descriptions, depending on who you ask. It's an approach to psychology that focuses on the positive. This means the principles revolve around creating a good, happy life instead of getting held back by trying to fix the bad parts. The concept isn't to ignore human struggles or the presence of bad things and problems. Instead, the aim is to emphasize the good so that struggles can be overcome and the positive can outshine the negative to foster resilience. To build a life in which we can truly flourish, we need to:

- Prioritize positive emotions instead of dwelling on the negative feelings
- Acknowledge achievements instead of focusing on what hasn't been achieved
- Cultivate strong and healthy relationships instead of trying to mend broken or unhealthy bonds

- Find ways to provide life with meaning

To do this, positive psychology uses a set of principles as a guideline for how to live life in a way that increases feelings of positivity and satisfaction. They're called PERMA Principles.

What are PERMA Principles?

PERMA is an acronym where each letter is associated with a concept that is meant to enhance positivity:

- Positive emotions
- Engagement
- Relationships (positive ones)
- Meaning
- Accomplishment

Let's look at each of these principles in more detail to better understand what they mean and how they encourage a positive psychological outlook on life.

Positive emotions: Experiencing feelings of happiness and positivity is crucial for mental wellbeing. Enjoyment, satisfaction, contentedness, and many other positive emotions can be experienced in various ways, such as fulfilling relationships, achieving goals, and doing things that bring pleasure. You can't be happy absolutely all the time, but you can prioritize that in life, which brings you happiness over the things that don't.

Engagement: Engagement can be experienced in different scenarios, such as in relationships or activities. The idea is that you're fully occupied or involved. You'll know the feeling of complete engagement if you've ever become so wrapped up in a conversation, activity, or experience that you lost track of time or were immune to regular distractions. You don't have to be totally absorbed in everything you do every moment of the day, but fully engaging from time to time is vital for a sense of wellbeing.

Relationships: Unlike bears, who prefer their own company, human beings tend to prefer the company of others. We're social creatures, and relationships are incredibly important to us. Relationships come in all shapes and sizes. Some are good for us, while others aren't. Purposely building strong, meaningful, and healthy relationships increases our sense of wellbeing, while superficial and unhealthy relationships or a lack of good relationships increases dissatisfaction.

Meaning: Finding meaning in life usually involves recognizing the world outside of ourselves and dedicating ourselves to a purpose that aligns with our personal values. Without meaning, you may feel listless and wonder, "What am I doing with my life?" or "Why am I here? What is my purpose?" Having meaning or purpose in one's life fosters a sense of wellbeing through feeling that your existence is validated and you're not just on this earth for no good reason.

Accomplishment: Accomplishment and achievement can be used interchangeably, and the terms mean different things to different people. What you consider an achievement might not feel like one to someone else and vice versa. Accomplishments or feelings of success are a driving force for happiness. Irrespective of your goals, the satisfaction gained from achievements fosters a sense of overall wellbeing.

How to use the PERMA Principles

Using the PERMA Principles in your own life to improve your psychological positivity and sense of wellbeing is actually easy.

- Positive emotions: Make time for the things that make you happy, whether activities or relationships.
- Engagement: Make time for the things you can become wholly engaged with, whether they're people or activities.
- Relationships: Purposely build positive relationships and prioritize spending time with those with whom you have positive relationships.
- Meaning: Dedicate your time and resources to a purpose or cause and you will feel your life has meaning.
- Accomplishment: Set goals and work on achieving them. Then, make mental space to acknowledge your accomplishments.

The problem with implementing these principles and pursuing lasting happiness is the misconception that it's an act of selfishness. Not everybody holds this opinion, but it does crop up more regularly than it should. From a young age, we're taught to be selfless, and a certain amount of self-lessness is healthy. However, society tends to go overboard with pushing the limits of selflessness. Consequently, when we don't conform to the ideas others have about how much we should be sacrificing our own wants and needs for others, we're labeled selfish. Taking a closer look at selfishness, the Merriam-Webster online dictionary defines selfishness as "concerned excessively or exclusively with oneself: seeking or concentrating on one's own advantage, pleasure, or wellbeing without regard for others" (Selfish, n.d.). Considering the definition, it's easy to see how prioritizing ourselves in any way, shape, or form is misconstrued as selfishness. The difference between being selfish and reasonably pursuing your happiness, wellbeing, and interests is whether you disregard others. When others are inconvenienced by your decisions, they'll automatically jump to the conclusion that you've heartlessly ignored their needs or wants. It will often be met with, "But what about me!?" This happens all the time. The moment someone isn't getting what they want from you because you are prioritizing yourself, you're the one being selfish. These same people don't, or won't, understand how their lack of consideration for you reverses the roles, making them the selfish party.

To put the importance of prioritizing your wellbeing into perspective, consider these two quotes:

"In order to care for others, you must care for yourself first." – Mary Scarpeti

"Taking care of myself doesn't mean 'me first'. It means 'me too'."– L. R. Knost.

Happiness and positivity are crucial for developing a sense of wellbeing. A sense of wellbeing is vital for your functioning as a healthy person and part of society. Without it, your ability to be productive and selfless when the opportunities arise is compromised. Implementing the PERMA principles in your daily and weekly life is paramount to your health, wellbeing, happiness, and success. If taking the time to do these things leads someone to call you out as "selfish", it's okay to reflect on whether or not you are genuinely disregarding them. If you're in doubt, remember the following quote and apply it to every situation that makes you question whether you really should be prioritizing yourself:

"When you say 'yes' to others, make sure you are not saying 'no' to yourself." – Paulo Coehlo.

Exercise: Reflection Questions

You may or may not already be applying PERMA Principles in your life. Even if you are implementing all of them, you may not be doing it in a balanced way to maximize a positive psychological state. Use these questions to help you create a more balanced approach to cultivating a positive mindset using PERMA.

- Which principles are you already applying in your life?

- Which principles are you overlooking and not applying?
- Which principles are your strong points? – Which ones are you good at applying?
- Which principles could you benefit from paying more attention to?
- How can you improve your application of the pertinent principles?

Simple Positive Psychology Tips

Invest in self-care: Self-care is anything you do to maintain or improve the wellbeing of your body and mind. Self-care looks different for everyone, but the outcome is the same; it increases happiness and satisfaction, reduces stress, and contributes to your health. Activities range from cooking nutritious meals or exercising to meditating, reading, listening to music, and much more.

Develop healthy coping skills: Stress is a constant shadow over modern life. You have to deal with regular, ever-present stressors, such as work, and acute, unforeseen situations that stir up powerful emotions quickly. Find ways that will help you effectively and constructively healthily deal with stress and emotions. Some coping skills may even overlap with self-care activities.

Take time to connect: Isolating yourself from your friends and family, even for short periods, can increase stress and unhappiness. No matter how busy your schedule is, be sure to take time to connect with the people you care about every week.

Talk it out: Keeping your thoughts and emotions to yourself could create a scenario where you feel like a human soda can that's been shaken, and you're about to explode. Talking about your feelings and thoughts, even the negative ones, is cathartic, and allows you to openly express yourself, and it improves communication between you and others, and can then lead to stronger relationships. Be mindful of being kind and considerate when giving voice to your negative emotions, in order to keep the communication healthy.

BUILDING MEANINGFUL RELATIONSHIPS

One of the PERMA Principles is to have healthy relationships. As social creatures, feeling connected or isolated from others can profoundly impact our health and wellbeing. Relationships form a vital part of our coping mechanisms to get us through tough times and mental and emotional hurdles such as anxiety and stress. These healthy connections create a support system that makes dealing with difficulties and living a healthy and happy life easier. You're more likely to make better choices supporting mental and physical health when you have a sense of social connectedness and solid, supportive relationships.

The thing about relationships is they're not always good for you. Not everybody gets along and has your best interests at heart. Relationships are also hard work, making it crucial to put effort into building and maintaining healthy relationships, whether romantic or platonic.

Growing up, we learn to navigate the potential minefield of social life and social interactions with others. Unfortunately, not many of us are taught how to identify healthy versus unhealthy relationships, or how to create connections that are good for us. As a result, many people build relationships lacking in certain areas or entertain connections with people who are toxic for their wellbeing. Any relationship is a two-way street, and the following fundamentals must be given and reciprocated to be healthy and beneficial for all involved.

Effective Communication

Communication is immensely significant in any relationship, and it goes far beyond being able to fluently speak a language. Effective communication is based on the 'seven Cs':

Clear: Whatever the message you are trying to get across, it must be clear and leave no room for assumption or misinterpretation.

Concise: The clarity of your message can easily get lost if you're too wordy or offer up too much information at once. Keep communication short, sweet, and to the point, to avoid confusion. Avoid using filler words or repeating the point using different phrasing.

Concrete: A concrete message is specific and clear, not vague, and provides the other person with all necessary information. Facts can be used to back up the message.

Correct: Try to make all message aspects accurate, from pronunciation and language use to spelling, grammar, facts, and names.

Complete: While you don't want to include too much information, you must have everything necessary and relevant to your message. Leaving out key details will leave room for confusion or assumptions, or you may fail to provide the other person enough information to understand what you're trying to tell them.

Coherent: Coherent communication includes all the relevant information for the discussed topic, and it is concise and correct, and doesn't veer off-topic. It's also delivered at a consistent speed and tone.

Courteous: For communication to be received well by others, it should be delivered using appropriate language and empathy. It should be open and honest while still being as kind as possible. Avoid passive-aggressive language, sarcasm, insults, a harsh tone, and other poor communication techniques that could interfere with how your message is received.

Active Listening

Active listening is a skill everyone can benefit from learning. It's a mindfulness technique that can increase the efficacy of your communication with others. Active listening allows you to remain in the moment, truly listen to the person speaking, absorb the information you're receiving, and stay grounded instead of letting your emotions run away with you. Use the following steps to start practicing active listening in your communication with others:

Listen: Truly listen to what is being said without getting distracted by other sights and sounds around you. Listen to the person's words with empathy. Try to put yourself in their shoes, as it were, to try to see the situation from their perspective.

Focus on the speaker, not your own thoughts: How often do you mentally formulate your response to someone while they are still talking? While you are working on your response, you aren't actually listening and taking on board what they are saying, and you're likely to miss crucial words, facts, or points they bring up.

Don't interrupt: Interrupting someone while they are speaking can derail their train of thought, change the topic, show you're formulating a response while you should be listening, and lead to a breakdown in communication.

Pay attention: True listening, not just hearing, requires you to give the speaker your full attention. Observe their body language for non-verbal cues and make appropriate eye contact. Smile and nod occasionally or use positive words of reinforcement, such as "yes" or "I see". Even if you don't like or disagree with what's being said, keep your own body language and expression neutral.

Clarify and question: Once the person has finished speaking, clarify what they said to ensure you understand correctly. Briefly summarize their key points, ask open-ended questions, and mention if there was anything you did not understand correctly. You can use phrasing such as "If I understand you correctly..." or "From my understanding, you're saying..." or "What do you mean when you say..."

Boundaries

Boundaries are rules within a relationship that each person sets, which outline how they want to be treated, to ensure they feel comfortable, safe, and respected. You don't have to like someone else's boundaries, and they don't have to like yours, but you do have to accept and respect each other's boundaries. Boundaries include what a person accepts in terms of others' behavior, what is expected of others, and how to express a person's personal limits. Here are a few tips for setting healthy boundaries in relationships:

- Communicate openly and honestly about what you need, want, and the limits in the relationship.
- Listen to the other person's wants, needs, and limits.
- Explain your boundaries clearly and concisely using the 'seven Cs' of effective communication.
- Express what the consequences of overstepping your boundaries will be.
- Avoid the temptation to apologize, justify, or make

excuses for your boundaries if the other person seems unhappy with them.

- Avoid requiring an apology or justification for the other person's boundaries.
- Be firm about your boundaries and mindful of not overstepping the boundaries of others.

Important note: Nobody goes into a relationship with all their boundaries in place from the start. It often takes time and many interactions to figure out what boundaries need to be set and when they should be employed. When discussing boundaries, especially after someone has overstepped without realizing it, do it calmly and courteously without allowing emotions to overrule your communication.

Emotional Expression

Expressing your emotions to others fosters a more profound connection by allowing yourself to trust someone with your vulnerability. It can be incredibly challenging because you are letting your guard down, which can lead to fear of getting hurt. It's usually easier to express positive emotions than negative ones, but bottling up hurt feelings and thoughts slowly poisons you from the inside. Here are some tips for healthily expressing your thoughts and feelings:

Take a step back: Immediately reacting to something upsetting generally means emotions are running high, and you haven't had time to reflect on your feelings. Take time to "cool off" and understand your emotions before bringing them up with the other person.

Label and understand your emotions: Identify your feelings and why you feel the way you do. Sometimes, emotions don't stem from what initially seems to trigger them. You could feel irritated or angered by someone's words or actions because you're tired or stressed, and not because of what was actually said or done.

Consider the repercussions: Sometimes, we can deal with our emotions ourselves without bringing them up to others. Consider what you're feeling, where those emotions genuinely come from, and whether it's necessary to share them or if sharing them will only result in a negative outcome.

Time your expression appropriately: Discussing emotions can be a sensitive exercise, and timing plays a massive role in how well the discussion goes. Ask yourself whether you are in the correct headspace to have a productive talk, and ask the other person whether it's a good time for them to chat about your feelings. If there is a better time for one of you, work out when would be better for the conversation.

Use "I feel..." statements: Whenever you begin a statement with "I feel...", you are prioritizing your feelings over the situation. When you start with "When you...", the statement comes across as attacking, which may make the other person go on the defensive instead of listening to you and opens the door for the conversation to deteriorate into an argument.

Use the seven Cs of effective communication and active listening: Throughout a meaningful conversation about emotions, follow the seven Cs to ensure your message is conveyed as best you can. When the other person has a turn to talk, employ active listening to facilitate a two-way discussion, not a one-way rant of your own.

Request changes mindfully: When someone has done or said something that truly upsets you, requesting a change or setting a boundary is vital. Do so in a kind but firm way by:

- Telling the person what you appreciate about them or what they're doing well in the relationship
- Expressing your feelings or concerns, why you feel that way, and how the other person can help avoid similar situations
- In the future, reminding the person that you care about them, value the relationship, and want to work on maintaining a meaningful connection with them

Check-in with each other: Regularly take time to connect with the people you care about and discuss feelings, expectations, and the relationship in general. This is especially important after a disagreement but is also a great way to talk about emotions and thoughts before they have time to fester and cause bigger issues.

Respect and Empathy

How you make someone feel will stick with them, even if they forget what you did or said to make them feel that way. Developing respect and empathy toward each other is critical for creating and maintaining a healthy relationship.

When you are respectful and empathetic, your interactions become easier, especially when dealing with conflict. Try these tips for being respectful and compassionate toward others:

- Communicate effectively without resorting to using foul or degrading language, laying blame, guilt-tripping, making excuses, making threats, or raising your voice.
- Listen actively.
- Don't disregard the other person's feelings or try to tell them how they should feel or what they should think.
- Put yourself in the other person's shoes to try to understand things from their perspective.
- Show others you appreciate them.
- Set and respect each other's boundaries.
- Express emotions in a healthy way.

Time

Spending time together is crucial for nurturing meaningful relationships, as is spending time apart. Set realistic expectations for how much time you are comfortable spending with each other and how much personal space and time apart is needed. When you're together, focus on connecting with each other and not just being in the same space. When you are apart, understand that no person can fulfill another person's every social and personal need, and time away from each other is healthy.

Differences and Change

Whether it's family, spouses, friends, or colleagues, expect there to be differences in values, opinions, thoughts, emotions, and much more. Not everybody will think, behave, or feel like you do, and that's okay. What's not okay is to expect others to change to conform to your expectations. There will, of course, be "deal-breakers" and differences that cannot be set aside. However, most of the time, the differences between people can be navigated respectfully to maintain the relationship. Many differences are minor, and some more pertinent ones can be overcome by agreeing to disagree, and by not holding the difference of opinion against each other. Where differences cause friction in the relationship, it's crucial to use effective communication, active listening, healthy emotional expression, respect, empathy, and compromise.

Accepting individual differences is vital for healthy connections. As is not expecting people to change to suit your preferences. However, that doesn't mean people don't change over time. As people mature and undergo personal growth, their values, thoughts, emotions, and behaviors may change. You should expect people to change as they develop throughout life, which may cause differences to arise. The relationship itself may change along with the people involved. As you notice changes in someone you care about, approach them with a discussion just as you would when dealing with differences. If the relationship changes or fizzles out, accept it as a part of life, and strive to continue building new healthy relationships instead of getting hung up on people who've drifted apart.

Trust and Privacy

Without trust, you cannot have a healthy relationship. Trust gives a person a sense of security and predictability when dealing with someone. A trustworthy person is viewed as safe, dependable, and credible. Trust is earned over time and by interacting with someone, and here's how you can build others' trust in you:

Keep your word, which means honoring your commitments and not making promises you cannot keep.

- Stick to your values and beliefs.
- Communicate openly and effectively.
- Listen actively.
- Be honest.
- Be kind and helpful without ulterior motives.
- Express your feelings to increase an emotional connection.
- Be humble and avoid 'blowing your own horn' or making things about yourself.
- Stand by personal boundaries and respect the boundaries of others.
- Freely admit any mistakes or wrongdoings and apologize sincerely.
- Be consistent in your actions and trust-building techniques.

Trust and privacy are inextricably linked. When you trust someone, you can give them privacy and you respect that privacy. When trust is lacking, suspicion creeps in, and the perception of privacy can become skewed into a desire to hide things. Privacy is vital in any relationship. It allows people to maintain an autonomous sense of self and avoid feeling smothered. Not having any privacy can lead to feelings of resentment and anger, so it's best to let people have their privacy, showing them you respect and trust them.

CULTIVATING AN ATTITUDE OF GRATITUDE

Gratitude is the ability to recognize, be thankful, and show appreciation for what you have in life. The power of cultivating gratitude includes the following:

- Gratitude encourages people to embrace and truly enjoy the present moment.
- Positive emotions are focused on and also magnified.
- Negative emotions that can cause mental and emotional distress, such as regret, resentment, and envy, are reduced.
- A person's sense of self-worth is buoyed.
- Gratitude breeds positivity, which, in turn, increases tolerance of stressors and resilience.

Considering all the good that comes from cultivating gratitude, you'd think everybody would jump on the bandwagon to tap into the benefits. However, gratitude can be challenging for some people, and here's why:

Being grateful can go against deeply ingrained beliefs, such as the human tendency for "self-serving bias". This psychological bias tells us that when we experience good things, it's because of our own efforts, but when we experience bad things, it's because of circumstances or other people. It allows us to take all the credit for the good in our lives and shift blame for the bad onto someone or something else. Gratitude opposes this because it requires us to share credit for the good in our lives by acknowledging the people who have helped us achieve our successes. Being grateful doesn't mean we have to hand over all the credit, as we did achieve success through our own efforts, but we can recognize that it wasn't all our own doing.

The second challenge to gratitude is the need for control. Being grateful encourages us to admit that things in life are beyond our control. The idea that we can't control our environment and not being omnipotent or understanding why everything happens can be pretty scary.

Lastly, gratitude doesn't allow us to indulge in the "just world" hypothesis. This idea encourages the belief that life is fair and we get what we deserve. The reality is very different. Good things can happen to bad people while bad things can also happen to good people. It's an aspect of life that cannot be explained, and gratitude encourages acceptance of all of this.

Exercise: Cultivating Gratitude

Gratitude can be built in various ways, and each person will find specific methods easier and more effective than others. Try out some of these techniques for cultivating gratitude to see which ones work for you.

Gratitude journaling: Spend a few minutes each day writing down at least three things you are grateful for in your life or your day.

Walk mindfully: Take a stroll to acknowledge and appreciate your surroundings. Take turns focusing on one of your senses at a time and finding things that you can see, hear, smell, and touch or feel.

Contemplate gratefully: Take a break from life and its distractions for 5-10 minutes, so no phones, TV, music, or anything else. Spend that time thinking of the good things you are thankful for.

Speak gratefully: Work on adding words and phrases of appreciation to your daily vocabulary when speaking to others, such as:

- I am grateful to/for you.
- I am indebted to you.
- I appreciate you.
- My sincere thanks.
- Thank you.
- Thanks.
- This is great.

- You are a blessing.
- You are a true friend.
- You are an inspiration.
- You light up my life.
- You make me happy.
- You're so great.
- You're the best.
- You've been very helpful.

Show gratitude: Make an effort to include expressions of your gratitude to others in your daily interactions with them. Learn which of the following five gratitude 'languages' suits a person best and show them you appreciate them by using their gratitude language to express your thankfulness:

- Use words or phrases of affirmation or give compliments.
- Give small, thoughtful gifts.
- Perform small acts of service or kindness.
- Give up your time and pay attention to the person.
- If appropriate, show appreciation through gentle physical touch like hugs, holding hands, and other signs of affection.

Use a gratitude reminder: Your aim is to increase your positivity. It's not going to happen overnight, and if you suffer from anxiety or persistent pessimistic thoughts, it can be hard to break the cycle of negativity. Carry an object in your pocket that will remind you to reflect on at least one thing you're grateful for every time you touch it.

USING POSITIVE AFFIRMATIONS

Positive affirmations can help reinforce gratitude, increase motivation, amplify positive emotions, and challenge negative thoughts. They're positive statements you can repeat to yourself when you need a positivity boost or to combat negative thoughts or feelings. The key to affirmations is to make an effort to believe what you are saying, rather than to merely parrot a positive sentence. Affirmations can be a powerful technique in your toolbox of positive psychology techniques. Studies have shown that affirmations can stimulate parts of the brain that encourage and increase the chances of making positive life changes (Peden, Rayens, & Hall, 2005).

Exercise: Writing an Affirmation Statement

You can easily write affirmation statements, tailoring them to your needs and wants. Follow these steps to write and use your own affirmation statements:

- Contemplate specific things or areas in your life you'd like to change. Ensure the changes align with your values and really matter to you to increase the efficacy of the affirmations.

- Base your affirmations on realistic and achievable goals. Affirmations must be believable, otherwise, you won't truly believe what you're telling yourself.
- Note negative thoughts or beliefs and create affirmations that are their positive opposite to repeat every time the negative thought occurs to you.
- Create affirmations in the present tense, not the future tense, to increase believability. For example, "I am confident." instead of "I will be confident."
- Use only positive wording in your affirmation. Avoid any negative phrasing. For example, "I am confident." instead of "I am not self-conscious."
- Say affirmations out loud and with feeling. Emotionally invest in the affirmation and inject feeling into your voice when you say it.

WHAT'S NEXT?

Your physical and mental health are inseparably linked to each other. To achieve true wellness, physical and mental approaches are necessary to address both sides of the gut-brain axis and its influence on your mind and body. You've discovered various strategies that can be employed to improve both. However, absorbing and implementing all of this information can feel like an overwhelming task. Where do you start, how do you go about making the necessary positive changes, what happens when you face challenges to a healthy lifestyle, and how do you maintain these changes for the foreseeable future?

In the next chapter, we will explore how to use what you have learned and the strategies you've discovered. We'll detail how to use this guide to implement healthy habits and tailor your gut health and mental wellness practices to suit your needs and personality. You'll discover common obstacles you could face and how to overcome them effectively. Finally, we'll discuss techniques to help you stay on track and cultivate lasting habits that will transform your life by improving your health.

6

PUTTING IT ALL TOGETHER

Throughout this guide, you've discovered how the gut and brain are interlinked. Connected by the microbe-gut-brain-axis communication channel, the gut is often casually thought of as the body's second brain. It also has various emotional and cognitive associations, from "gut feelings" to those fluttering "butterflies". However, the link and effect the gut and brain exert on each other extend further. Due to the communication between the two, if one is off-kilter, it can cause the other to experience disruptions. The gut-brain axis has far-reaching effects on overall health and wellbeing, making it crucial to adopt a lifestyle that equally supports gut health and mental wellness.

Stress is one of modern life's most significant factors that can impact the gut and brain. While stress is a natural and healthy response to certain threats to ensure survival, it can quickly become detrimental if not controlled. The human body isn't designed to maintain any level of stress response, or fight or flight mode, for extended periods. Stress is meant to be a short-lived periodic experience, not a frequent or chronic drain on our physical and mental resources. Prolonged elevated stress levels can wreak havoc on your physical and psychological wellbeing. Cortisol is a key culprit in this systemic lack of regulation. It throws appetite and eating habits out of balance, disrupts sleep, puts a damper on positivity, instigates low-grade body-wide inflammation, and skews crucial gut microbe population numbers, to name a few adverse effects. Stress exerts influence over mental and physical health, and the gut-brain axis compounds these symptoms by facilitating the impact the brain and gut have on each other.

While the gut-brain connection may seem like a problem by being able to exert a two-way negative influence on overall wellness, it can also do the complete opposite. You can use this bidirectional communication 'highway' to your advantage, prompting it to compound positive health outcomes in your favor. The trick is implementing positive lifestyle habits that bolster health and wellbeing at each connection. This guide provides you with a wide selection of practical and easily actionable habits that will help you transform your life by beneficially exploiting the gut-brain axis.

You can't just address the body's physical needs to achieve holistic wellbeing. Mental and emotional needs must also be met. You can do all the physically correct things to achieve a healthy lifestyle, such as ensuring your diet is balanced and nutritious and getting enough exercise. However, if you're not caring for your mental and emotional wellbeing, the gut-brain axis will allow an unhappy mind to detract from your body's wellness. When the body's health then declines, the mind can suffer even more, and this could lead to a cycle of overall physical and mental health deterioration. This cycle may leave you vulnerable to anxiety and even depression, two mental health obstacles that feed off each other.

Using the knowledge gained in this guide, you can successfully and effectively transform your lifestyle to support optimal health and wellness. The only potential hurdle is not knowing where to start or how to tailor the program to your preferences. Evaluating your lifestyle and coming to the realization that there are many new habits you need to incorporate can seem overwhelming. You may also notice we've not laid out a predetermined, sequentially structured step-by-step process. Of course, the guide can be followed sequentially, starting with part one and ending with part four. However, that doesn't necessarily have to be the case. You can just as easily and effectively start with whichever part you want to begin with or even pick out strategies from each part to implement simultaneously. How you use this guide to boost your gut health and mental wellness is entirely up to you.

Overhauling an unhealthy lifestyle takes time and isn't a process that is applied in the way for everyone. There is no right or wrong place to start. The decision on where to start and what to change first is profoundly personal and can affect your overall success. Your success will depend on how you reflect on your life, the changes you want to make, and your own personality to tailor the program to your needs. How quickly you adopt these changes will also have a great effect on the success of your wellness journey. The guide is split into four parts, but that doesn't mean you have to start with part one and end with part four. You don't even have to focus on one part at a time until you've mastered it before moving on to another one. You could pick out practices from each part to implement at the same time. How you use this guide is entirely up to you, but here are some helpful suggestions you may wish to consider:

- If you want to focus on one part at a time, pick the part that will be easiest to master. This can help build your confidence, motivation, and determination by presenting the fewest challenges, and the obstacles that will be the easiest to overcome.
- If you want to start including practices from different parts simultaneously, pick habits or changes that will be easiest to implement and maintain. Work your way up to more difficult changes to help keep up your motivation and confidence.
- Avoid making too many changes at one time.
- Prioritize the areas of your lifestyle that are the most important to change, and start with the practices that will most significantly impact in those areas.

- If there are changes that require resources you don't yet have, start with the changes you do have the resources for and revisit other practices later when you are ready.
- Find support. Nobody can make your lifestyle changes for you, but they can support you along the way by improving your accountability, buoying your motivation, and offering a source of advice or reassurance when you face setbacks or challenges.

MAINTAINING GUT HEALTH AND MENTAL WELLNESS

The truth about lasting change is that it all starts in your mind. Irrespective of what kind of change you're trying to make, if you don't change the way you think, it's not going to stick. No amount of trying to force, reward, punish, or otherwise coerce yourself into making that change, and maintaining it, will be productive without first making a mental shift.

Your thoughts influence your behavior and your emotions. You are always going to feel resistant to change if your thoughts about it stay the same, and over time, that inner resistance will chip away at your motivation and determination. Eventually, old behaviors creep back in, and change is abandoned. Many of the thoughts that prevent you from making lasting lifestyle changes stem from your core beliefs. Core beliefs are strong beliefs a person has about themselves, other people, and the world around them. They're deeply ingrained in the subconscious, and while they give rise to a variety of "surface" thoughts, many people don't realize what their core beliefs are and how they impact their lives.

So many people are held back by their beliefs, and you may have even fallen victim to deeply rooted self-limiting assumptions in the past. These beliefs are incredibly powerful but also very fragile at the same time. You see, they're often not based on incontestable proof or fact. They're merely assumptions. As much power as your beliefs have to influence your behavior, the good news is that you have just as much control over changing them. It takes time and consistent effort, but don't let that put you off trying. Here's how your beliefs influence achieving true change and why you should work on changing some of them.

- Negative core beliefs are like magnets. They attract any shred of negativity that could possibly relate to them and repel any form of positivity that could undermine them.
- Negative core beliefs cause your mind to focus on perceived negatives and may even emphasize them, making them seem more unpleasant than they really are.
- Negative core beliefs produce automatic negative thoughts (ANTs), which are thoughts that pop into your head automatically without giving you time to consider how factual they are.
- ANTs support negative core beliefs and may foster self-doubt.

- When combined, negative beliefs, their ANTs, and the resulting self-doubt can reduce the amount of effort you put into making lifestyle changes stick.
- When you don't give something your all, the risk of failing is increased, and progress toward achieving a goal can be slowed down.
- Slow progress toward success or even struggling to overcome challenges along the way due to not putting in maximum effort might be acting as affirmations of your self-doubt. Self-doubt feeds negative beliefs, and your mind uses the slower progress and setbacks as "proof" that the beliefs are, in fact, true.
- When your beliefs have you wholly convinced that something is too difficult and you just can't do it, you're left wide open to throwing in the towel and giving up. When you do, that deep-seated core belief smirks and says, "I told you so!"

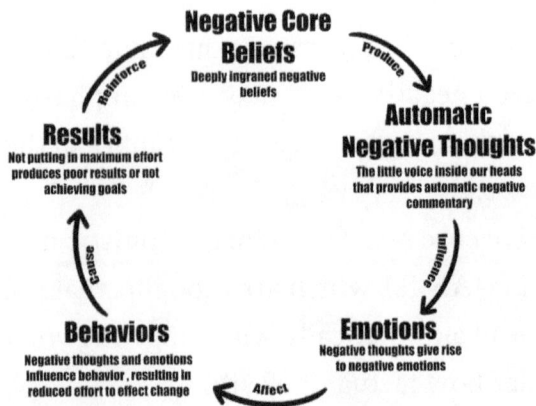

Negative Core Beliefs
Deeply ingraned negative beliefs

Automatic Negative Thoughts
The little voice inside our heads that provides automatic negative commentary

Emotions
Negative thoughts give rise to negative emotions

Behaviors
Negative thoughts and emotions influence behavior, resulting in reduced effort to effect change

Results
Not putting in maximum effort produces poor results or not achieving goals

Exercise: Changing Negative Beliefs

Core beliefs are so deep and often long-standing that changing them can be difficult, especially when strong emotions are attached to them. These changes also don't happen overnight, which is another reason many people find it particularly hard to do. However, with consistency, rewiring the way you think can be achieved. The following steps will help you identify and change negative thoughts and beliefs.

Step One: Identify Automatic Negative Thoughts

For a week or two, whenever a negative thought about the lifestyle change you're trying to make pops into your head, write the following details down:

- The thought
- The date of the thought
- The time of the thought
- The circumstances: what happened that gave rise to the ANT?
- Your emotions: list at least one emotion the ANT made you feel
- Your response to the thought: how did you react to the thought and the resulting emotions, or how did they influence your behavior?

Step Two: Challenge and Replace ANTs

You can do step two immediately after step one, or you can schedule time later in the day to do it, but the sooner after the thought, the better. Think about the ANT free from judgment about yourself, others, or the world around you. Look at it as if it were something detached from you without allowing prejudice or bias from your hidden core beliefs to take over. Now, answer these questions:

- Is the thought rooted in an opinion or an assumption, or is it based on fact?
- If the thought is rooted in an opinion or an assumption, is there evidence to prove, beyond a reasonable doubt, that it's correct?
- How did you come to this opinion or assumption? Where does it come from, and why do you believe it?
- Is the opinion or assumption helpful or harmful to you? Does the belief make you happy or help you progress toward your goals, or does it make you unhappy or hinder your progress?
- What is a positive or helpful thought you can replace the ANT with, thereby challenging the negative thinking and adapting your beliefs to a more productive perspective?

Step 3: Anticipate ANTs

Automatic negative thoughts are, as the name implies, automatic, but they often crop up in response to a situation. Learning to anticipate the circumstances that prompt ANTs allows you to catch them more easily and challenge them more effectively. Use these tips for anticipating ANTs.

- Become aware of your ANTs and the circumstances that provoke them.
- Be mindful of your surroundings, interactions with others, and activities.
- If you find yourself in a situation or think you may encounter a situation that triggers an ANT, mentally prepare for it by planning what positive thought to replace the negative one with.
- If your ANTs are linked to strong emotional responses, have appropriate, effective coping strategies ready to help manage your emotions when they are stirred up.
- Be consistent with challenging your ANTs. Without making excuses, challenge them every single time.

MENTAL AND EMOTIONAL OBSTACLES TO EFFECTIVE CHANGE

Challenging and overcoming unhelpful core beliefs and automatic negative thoughts is only one way of effecting lasting mental health lifestyle changes. Even when you tackle your negative thoughts and improve your mental attitude toward change, and your ability to achieve success, other roadblocks may appear. Here are three common mental and emotional obstacles that can trip you up along your journey and how to deal with them.

All-or-Nothing Thinking

This is a mentality so many people have and don't even realize how bad it is for them. With this type of thinking, it's all in or all out. There are no stepping stones to get to where they want to be and no in-between. Other terms to describe this kind of thinking include "black or white" thinking or the saying, "Go big or go home."

The problem with all-or-nothing thinking is that it's more often than not hugely impractical. Life isn't just black and white, there are many gray areas and many different hues of gray. Similarly, very little in life is ever achieved by approaching a challenge with the idea that you have to go flat out from the start or not do it at all. Usually, we don't have the resources necessary to go all-in from the get-go, whether that's time, energy, physical ability, or anything else.

All-or-nothing thinking puts you in a position that's high risk, and you are likely to give up if you either can't adhere to large-scale changes across the board or if you slip up at any time. Instead, you should aim to cultivate a progressive achievement mindset that allows you to start slow and build up to your ultimate goal. This approach also facilitates self-forgiveness when mistakes happen.

Exercise: Practice the 80/20 Rule

Economist Vilfredo Pareto discovered a trend in the late 19th century. His observations picked up the tendency for 80% of outcomes to be generated by 20% of the input (Guy-Evans, 2023). The concept was nicknamed the eighty-twenty rule. This framework can also be applied to a healthy lifestyle whereby you live healthily 80% of the time and can indulge in less healthy habits 20% of the time. This rule can be applied in a myriad of ways to suit your personal needs, such as:

- Making 80% of your daily diet super healthy while 20% isn't as healthy
- Having a "cheat" or "rest" day weekly
- Working out at moderate to high intensity 80% of the time and low intensity 20% of the time

These are just a few ideas, but there are so many options for implementing the 80/20 rule. Get creative and find a way to use it that fits your lifestyle and goals.

Comparison Thinking

Do you often compare yourself to others? You may be stuck in a comparison mindset. Making comparisons between yourself and others is normal and can be healthy, up to a point. It can, however, become problematic if you overdo it, or if you do it in the wrong way. Yes, there is a right and a wrong way to make comparisons.

Comparing oneself to another person is called social comparison. Human beings have an innate drive to make these comparisons as a way to more accurately perform self-evaluations. Others become the proverbial yardstick to measure how we stack up in an area of our lives. It's not common to compare one's entire being to the entire being of another but rather to focus on specific factors. There are two kinds of social comparisons, namely upward and downward. Each comes with benefits and drawbacks, and both can become unhealthy if done too often or too intensely.

Upward comparisons happen when we compare ourselves to someone we admire or perceive to be better than us. This can be a useful comparison to make if done correctly to boost motivation for self-improvement. Downward comparisons happen when we compare ourselves to people we perceive as not being as good as us. The theory behind downward comparisons is that they provide a form of self-protection when we're in a place of mental or emotional distress, as well as a way to boost self-confidence. Both types of comparisons can be detrimental, but upward comparison is especially risky as it can lead to deterioration in self-worth.

Often, comparison thinking doesn't take a person's uniqueness into account. This blindness to crucial individual differences is compounded by the social construct that aims to convince you that if one person can do something, anyone can do it. Phrases that demonstrate this fundamentally flawed concept include, "If I can do it, anyone can, and so can you." or "If so-and-so can do it, so can I." The problem is everyone is different and, as such, is capable of different things. Many factors affect what is and isn't possible for any one person, including genetics, upbringing, mental and emotional state, IQ, age, and physical health.

Comparisons should only be made against people who are as similar to us as possible to ensure our goals are actually attainable. Furthermore, comparisons should be done from a pragmatic point of view, not an emotionally-fueled subjective one. For example, someone who is genetically predisposed to be bigger-boned or voluptuous shouldn't compare themselves to someone who is naturally waif-like. The comparison should be made against someone with a similar body type or genetics. The comparison should also be made against someone with a similar body type with the view to become healthier, fitter, or a better person, and not for social acceptance or due to peer pressure. It should also not be an all-consuming thought that turns into an obsession or compulsion because even people with similar body types are fundamentally different from one another in many other ways.

Exercise: Combat Comparison Thinking

To combat comparison thinking can be hard, especially when we're bombarded with so many stimuli through media such as the internet, TV, movies, advertisements, social media, and more. Curbing a tendency to make unhelpful or unhealthy comparisons involves several elements:

Trigger avoidance: Comparisons can be made at anytime, anywhere, and against anyone. However, it's more often the case that they happen in response to triggers. Think about what usually triggers you to compare yourself to others. It may be you are triggered by certain social media accounts, particular people, or specific situations. Figure out what your comparison triggers are so you can avoid them when possible. If you can, replace negative triggers with positive ones. For example, unfollow social media accounts that make you feel bad about yourself and follow ones that make you feel more positive.

Gratitude: Gratitude is a powerful tool for redirecting your energy from a negative direction into a positive one. Each time you find yourself feeling or thinking negatively as a result of comparing yourself to someone else, practice gratitude. Think about three things you are grateful for about yourself, and why you're grateful for them. Even better yet, write down what you're grateful for to increase your focus on the positive aspects of your life.

Achievement Focus: Whether it's improving your health, advancing your career, getting fitter, or any other goal you are working toward, reflect on your achievements so far. When a negative comparison starts to creep in, remind yourself of where you started, your accomplishments to date, and the progress you've made toward your goals. To help you truly focus on your achievements, use progress measurements, such as photos, to drive the message of your success home and drown out the unhelpful comparison.

Impatience

It's no secret that we live in a world of increasing instant gratification. There are so many factors that contribute to our modern culture of impatience, from parenting to stress to the internet, and it's almost become ingrained in us as a norm. The good news is that it's a habit, and habits can be changed. Learning patience is vital for improving your chances of making long-term lifestyle changes stick and decreasing your risk of giving up. It can also help challenge and overcome negative beliefs and automatic negative thoughts.

Exercise: Improve Your Patience

Use these tips in different situations to help you learn to be more patient with yourself, the progress you are making, and the process of lifestyle change.

Understand: Despite the number of "achieve success quickly" advertisements and online posts you see, the truth is change takes time. Whether you are trying to lose weight, get fitter, or see the health results of your lifestyle changes, it's going to take time. You need to truly grasp this concept to be able to put the brakes on your impatience. Try reminding yourself that anything worth achieving is worth working for, and quick fixes don't last. Further, remind yourself of Aesop's fable of the tortoise and the hare , which teaches us that "Slow and steady wins the race."

Reframe: Often, impatience with a situation can be traced back to a source. Think about why you are being impatient and try to reframe the issue more positively. For example, you may want to lose weight or get fitter more quickly because of societal pressure. That is a mentally and emotionally unhelpful reason. If your reason for being impatient isn't helpful to your long-term wellbeing, reframe the situation. You could shift your focus from the pressure you're feeling, to the long-term health benefits of making the lifestyle change, or replace the idea of changing for others with the motivation of changing for yourself.

Get uncomfortable: Impatience can often stem from feeling uncomfortable, and nobody actively likes feeling uncomfortable. Learning to deal with uncomfortable feelings physically, mentally, and emotionally removes the drive for immediate results in order to escape the discomfort. Discomfort is unpleasant and makes your mind focus on the fact that you are not happy with the current state of things. Refocus your attention on the benefits you will gain as you make progress toward your goals.

THE ROLE OF ACCOUNTABILITY

Accountability has become somewhat of a buzzword in the modern world as more people realize just how vital a life skill it is. Accountability is the ability to accept responsibility for your own actions. At its core, accountability comes down to rejecting the temptation to make excuses, no matter how uncomfortable accepting responsibility for your actions may be. One thing accountability is not; it's not beating yourself up over making mistakes. Rather, it's a mental attitude that supports acceptance of your responsibilities to yourself, self-reflection on past behavior to improve in the future, and striving for success. Admitting your flaws or mistakes can seem counterproductive for motivation, but it's the exact opposite. Doing away with excuses that keep you stuck in a rut can improve motivation to put maximum effort into becoming a better, healthier, happier you.

For example, You could be adopting a healthier diet, and on the day you scheduled meal preparation time for the week ahead, friends or family drop by unannounced, taking up your usual meal preparation time. As a result, you end up opting for convenience foods during the week, derailing your healthy eating efforts. There are two ways to approach this scenario:

- **Lacking accountability:** Your response to not eating healthfully for a week would be something like, "I couldn't eat healthily this week because I didn't have time to prepare the meal."
- **Taking accountability:** Your response to not eating healthfully for a week would be something like, "I didn't eat healthily this week because I chose not to make time to prepare the meals or investigate quick healthy recipes for each night."

Exercise: Developing Accountability

The great thing about accountability is that it can be learned. Making excuses is a habit people learn at a young age to avoid the discomfort of owning up to their actions and dealing with the consequences of negative actions. As with any habit, shirking responsibility for one's own actions through excuses can be unlearned and replaced with the positive habit of taking accountability. Here's how to do it:

Step 1: Identify Your Personal Responsibilities

There are things you are responsible for and things you aren't. You are responsible for your own thoughts, emotions, words, and actions. You are not, however, responsible for the thoughts, emotions, words, or actions of others.

For example:

- You are responsible for challenging and changing negative or unhelpful thoughts, opinions, or views you hold to create a more positive and helpful mental state. You are not responsible for what others think about anything. Your actions or words may influence someone else's thoughts on a matter, but you cannot control what their thoughts are.
- You are responsible for your own emotions and learning effective emotional regulation and coping strategies for dealing with negative emotions. You are not responsible for how anyone else feels about anything. Your actions or words can evoke emotion from others, but you cannot control what emotions they feel.
- You are responsible for what you say and for controlling your verbal interactions with others, so

that your words don't cause justifiable offense, negative thoughts, or emotional pain to them. You are not responsible for the words that come out of anyone else's mouth. Your words can influence the thoughts and emotions of others, but you cannot control what they think or feel.

- You are responsible for your own actions and for controlling your behavior so that you don't cause unjustifiable offense, negative thoughts, or emotional pain to others. You cannot control anyone else's behavior. Your behavior can influence the thoughts and emotions of others, but again, you can't control what they think or feel.

Now, to think to yourself "I can't control what someone else thinks, feels, says, or does." might initially seem like a cop-out in a way. The thought can easily be used to excuse your own actions or words, to remove personal accountability, based on the idea that if your words or actions upset someone else, that's their problem because you can't control what they think or feel. This is where mindfulness, kindness, compassion, and empathy come into play. You are responsible for behaving and speaking to other people in a way that does not intentionally cause them to think or feel negatively. If you unintentionally cause someone to have negative thoughts or emotions, it's your responsibility to acknowledge their thoughts, feelings, and reactions, discuss the matter, apologize if their thoughts and emotions are reasonable, and make an effort not to repeat the situation in the future. If your words or actions do not reasonably justify a negative response, it's not your responsibility to manage anyone else's reaction. It is their responsibility to take personal accountability, as explained above, to navigate the situation in a positive way instead of in a negative, unhelpful manner.

Ultimately, you are responsible for yourself, and being accountable entails you avoiding making excuses where a reasonable alternative is an option. However, if something happens that is out of your control without a reasonable alternative course of action on your behalf, you're not responsible.

Step 2: Have an Action Plan

This ties in with identifying what you are responsible for. When adopting a holistically healthy lifestyle, you are responsible for implementing the changes necessary to become healthier. If you don't set goals and create a plan for achieving them, you aren't able to identify what actions you are responsible for. We will delve into setting SMART goals and creating a blueprint for success a bit later in the chapter. However, it's imperative to understand that without goals and a plan to do what you need to in order to reach them, it's extremely easy to find an excuse for a lack of progress. If you don't know where you want to be or what you need to do to get there, how can you hold yourself responsible for taking the necessary steps to arrive at your destination?

Step 3: Cultivate Brutal Honesty

Honesty is the enemy of an excuse. Bending the truth or lying outright to yourself in order to convince yourself that your thoughts, emotions, words, or actions are out of your control, negates taking accountability. Being completely honest with yourself can be a bitter pill to swallow. The ramifications of taking personal accountability often come to bite us after our actions and make us reflect on why we didn't make a better choice at the moment. Honesty means acknowledging you could have made a better choice and allows you to change your decision-making process in the future.

Step 4: Apologize

When poor decisions are made, apologies are necessary. Sometimes, you need to apologize to someone else so you can make amends and maintain a healthy relationship. Other times, you need to apologize to yourself so you can move past a mistake and do better in the future instead of getting sucked into a cycle of beating yourself up over it. Personal apologies and self-forgiveness prevent you from holding onto past mistakes which would otherwise tear down your self-worth, deflate your motivation, and keep you from achieving your goals.

Step 5: Learn to Manage Your Time

Time management helps you to budget every precious moment of your day to maximize what you get out of life.

Learning proper time management doesn't mean you have to turn into an inflexible, controlling tyrant. It means identifying priorities and planning your time to make sure your priorities are taken care of in order of importance. Here are some of the basic principles of daily time management:

- Prioritize: Dedicate time to doing what is most urgent before making time for less important activities.
- Plan: Consider how long activities will take, realistically, and allocate an appropriate amount of time for each activity or task.
- Expect the unexpected: Things don't always go according to plan. If something unexpected comes up, look at ways to adjust your daily schedule to maximize productivity.
- Don't delay: The old adage "Don't put off until tomorrow what you can do today," is a great life lesson. You never know what tomorrow holds or when something unexpected will pop up. If you have the time and resources to do something today, even if it could wait till tomorrow, you'll lessen your stress and make the most of your time if you act in the present.
- Create routines: Routines are the basis for picking up new, good habits. That's not to say you should be inflexible or only do the exact same things at the exact same time each day. Routines foster a sense of

familiarity, predictability, and responsibility. They can be rigidly structured, such as taking medication at a certain time every day, or they can be flexible, such as performing certain tasks in sequence so each previous task acts as a cue to do the next.

- Minimize distractions: Distractions take up your precious time needlessly. Have you ever noticed how checking one notification leads to checking others until you've spent half an hour checking unnecessary notifications? Similarly, you may have previously found yourself sucked into endless social media or news article scrolling. Giving in to a distraction for one moment can lead to minutes, if not hours, of lost time. Identify your common distractions and find ways to minimize them.

Step 6: Don't Over Commit

Piling too much on your plate daily, weekly, or monthly is a recipe for disaster. Juggling work, home life, social life, and personal goals can be tricky. Just because you are certain you have the time and resources to accomplish something, it does not mean you should commit to it. We often over-commit due to pressure or wanting to please others but end up disappointing ourselves and others when we can't pull through. Not being able to meet all our responsibilities also ramps up our stress levels. Understanding what your capabilities and limitations are, and learning to say no, will go a long way to avoiding the over-commitment trap.

SET SMART GOALS

SMART is a guideline that allows you to set goals that align with realistic expectations of yourself and your circumstances. It also helps build a foundation for creating an action plan for achieving your goals. SMART goals are:

Specific: A vague goal doesn't give you a clear endpoint to aim for, nor does it help you clearly plan how to achieve it. To announce, "I want to adopt a healthier diet," doesn't give you much clarity on the endpoint, how to measure progress, or how to achieve the goal. The statement, "I want to eat a balanced diet where 80% of my meals are 45% non-starchy veggies, 20% starch, 25% protein, and 10% fat," on the other hand, provides clarity on what percentage of your diet will be healthy and what healthy, balanced meals look like.

Measurable: If you can't measure progress toward a goal, you won't know when you've achieved it or be able to boost motivation by reflecting on how far you've already come. You can't tell whether you are really eating healthily or not. Furthermore, you won't know where you are in your diet transformation by just stating, "I want to adopt a healthier diet." You can, however, measure your progress toward eating healthily more often, and you can gauge how healthy your meals are, when you state, "I want to eat a balanced diet where 80% of my meals are 45% non-starchy veggies, 20% starch, 25% protein, and 10% fat."

Achievable: Everyone has fallen into the trap of aiming for an unattainable goal at some point in their lives. Unachievable goals are self-sabotaging, reinforcing negative beliefs, and tearing down your motivation. The attainability of a goal refers to the goal itself and the timeframe you give yourself to reach it. Setting achievable goals doesn't mean you can't aim high or that you should keep the bar low. It just means your goals should be realistic.

Relevant: A goal should be relevant to your values. Setting a goal that doesn't align with your values deflates your motivation to achieve it. Aiming to adopt a healthier diet because someone said you eat too much junk food, if you don't actually care about the opinions of others, isn't going to push you to achieve it. Aiming to adopt a healthier diet because it's important to you to live a long and actively involved life is more likely to motivate you to make your new diet stick.

Time-bound: Having a clear idea of what you want to achieve isn't going to do very much if you don't set a realistic time limit for achieving it. Without a deadline, you could spend years, if not decades, not really making much progress because there's no sense of urgency.

Exercise: Setting SMART Goals with a Mission Statement

A mission statement is a useful way to set a SMART goal and improve motivation. It's not your blueprint for reaching your goal and doesn't include the steps you will take to get there. It's simply a short statement, a personal promise to yourself, that outlines your goal using the SMART principles. Use the following example as a template for writing your own mission statement.

"I, (your name), promise myself that I will (clearly specify your goal in detail) by (set a clear, realistic deadline for achieving your goal). I want to (briefly summarize your goal) because (clearly detail your reasons for wanting to achieve the goal, be specific, and ensure the reasons are supported by your values). I am going to check in with myself (insert intervals for progress checks) and measure my progress toward achieving my goal by (insert how you'll measure your progress). I am responsible for putting in the effort to get what I want out of life, and I will hold myself accountable for reaching my goal."

Tip: If you ever need motivation quickly to spur on your determination when your commitment to your goal seems to be wavering, take out your mission statement and read it again.

CREATE A PLAN OF ACTION

When it comes to reaching any goal, you can't just go about it unprepared. That's a bit like saying you want to go to a specific town without detailed navigation instructions, hitting the road in the general direction of that town, and hoping for the best. You risk delays reaching your destination, getting lost, or not arriving at all. Your plan for reaching your goals is your roadmap to success. The advantages of creating a detailed blueprint for attaining your goals include:

Efficacy: It's nearly impossible to be effective at anything if you don't know what you are doing. Implementing the necessary changes to improve your lifestyle will be easier to do and keep track of for monitoring your progress.

Accountability: Holding yourself to account is a huge part of making any change yourself. Yet you can't hold yourself accountable for failing to take the necessary steps toward your goal if you don't know what those steps are. Having a clear understanding of what changes need to be made, how you're going to make them, and when you're going to implement them, makes personal accountability much easier.

Avoiding procrastination: By putting off doing what needs to be done you may slow your progress, or lower your motivation, and you will increase your risk of giving up. Not planning your path to your end goal encourages indecisiveness and procrastination. Having a solid plan minimizes unnecessary decision-making that could slow you down or trip you up along the way. Questions about what to eat or what exercise to do on any given day are answered well in advance, freeing you to get on with what you need to do instead of wasting time trying to make in-the-moment choices.

Exercise: Tailoring Your Action Plan

Each person is unique and, therefore, requires an individual plan for achieving their goals. Looking at how others achieve similar goals can serve as inspiration for your own action plan, but you don't have to copy what others do down to the letter. It's crucial to tailor your plan to your personal preferences, circumstances, capabilities, aspirations, and needs. Here are some tips for customizing your steps to success:

Meal planning: As previously discussed, meal planning and prepping is a fantastic way to save time and take the stress out of maintaining a healthy diet even if your schedule is quite hectic. Make sure to try new recipes as well as your favorite foods and that your planned meals cater to your particular dietary or nutritional goals.

Fitness planning: Not all physical activity is of equal value to an individual. Various types of exercise produce different results. Pick an exercise that will help you reach your particular fitness or physical goals and choose activities you actually enjoy. Plan to exercise on days of the week that suit you and at a time in the day when you feel you enjoy and benefit from it the most.

Stress management: Stress can have profound negative effects on your physical and mental health. It's vital to include stress management strategies in your plan to ensure you are adopting a holistic approach. Without practicing effective stress mitigation and management strategies regularly, you could be undermining your motivation and determination to stick to your lifestyle goals. When you're not in the right mental space, even the best of intentions could fall by the wayside.

TIPS FOR MAINTAINING YOUR MOTIVATION

Motivation is a key aspect of achieving any goal. The more motivated you are, the more effort you're likely to put into reaching a goal. However, motivation to keep working toward your desires, no matter how much you want them, can and does fluctuate. Your motivation can vary depending on your mood, stress levels, how busy you are, and many other factors. Try some of these tips for maintaining motivation when you feel your drive to succeed is running low:

Create a vision board: A vision board is a visual representation of your goal. Create a collage of inspirational images relating to your goal that you can look at to remind yourself what you are working toward.

Visualize your success: Visualization can be incredibly powerful if you commit to really applying your imagination. Envision yourself as having reached your goal and really try to experience it in your mind's eye. Include aspects of your success that will make the vision come alive inside you, such as how it will feel emotionally. It can take some practice but work on honing your focus to really put yourself in that position.

Affirm yourself: Create your own affirmations that will make you feel motivated using the exercise in the previous chapter. Tailor the affirmations to encourage motivation and help you overcome setbacks or obstacles.

Get support: Sometimes, we need a little help staying motivated, and that's where building relationships with like-minded people can be useful. From workout buddies to online support groups, interacting with people with similar values and goals can keep you going when your motivation is running low.

Track your progress: Change typically takes time. Depending on your goal, your journey could last weeks, months, or even years. During this time, you can easily lose sight of how much progress you've made. Track your progress using a journal, photos, measurements, old clothes, or whatever you feel helps you keep a clear picture of where you started and how far you've come. When your motivation falters, turn to your progress tracking to remind yourself of your success so far.

Find non-food rewards: Food is often used as a reward, starting from a young age. This is a surefire way to develop or perpetuate an unhealthy relationship with food. Find meaningful rewards you can treat yourself with when you achieve goals, and don't forget to celebrate smaller goals as well as the bigger ones.

Love and be kind to yourself: Nothing depletes motivation like self-deprecation and focusing on setbacks. Take time to show yourself some love and be kind to yourself, especially after a setback or when you're finding it hard to stick to your lifestyle changes. You don't have to excuse your mistakes or relapse into bad habits. Maintain accountability but speak to yourself kindly and forgive yourself so you can move past disappointment, in order to continue striving for success.

PRACTICE THE PRINCIPLES OF POSITIVE HOLISTIC WELLBEING BY SPREADING AWARENESS

Wellbeing is like a jigsaw puzzle. You can only enjoy it in its entirety when all the pieces have been put in place, and you can see the whole picture. Each piece of your wellness puzzle is a facet that contributes to the overall image being created. This includes facets such as emotions, mental space, and physical health, and each area is made up of several pieces.

Positivity forms a significant part of your mental health which is integral to your holistic wellness. There are many ways to incorporate positivity into your life. Some simple yet effective ways to do that are through sharing, kindness, and helping others. Sharing and helping others can boost your own mental wellness by reducing stress levels, improving mood, increasing feelings of confidence and self-esteem, and by enhancing feelings of happiness.

If you have found value in this guide and are enjoying the benefits of the knowledge you've gained, why not inject some positivity into your day by tapping into the mental wellness effects of sharing and helping others? By spreading awareness of the benefits and value you've gained from reading and working through this guide, you can help bring others' attention to the principles of a gut health and mental wellness-oriented lifestyle. To do this, you don't have to go out and start shouting about it from the mountaintops. **One way you can do this is to leave an honest and helpful review that will increase the visibility of this guide and let others know how helpful you found the information provided.**

Please visit the link below or scan the QR code to leave feedback on Amazon.

https://www.amazon.com/review/create-review/?asin=1738431223

CONCLUSION

As this guide comes to an end, take a moment to marvel at the intricate relationship between our gut and our brain. The gut-brain axis is more than just a physiological link between the mental and the physical. It's a powerful symbiosis that brings two essential organs together to govern our overall health. Even more than that, we can now appreciate that the gut isn't just an organ. It's a vibrant ecosystem, teeming with microscopic life, and despite their diminutive size, these tiny microbes have the power to influence our physical wellbeing, thoughts, and feelings. It's a microscopic world we're not consciously aware of, but it affects every part of our physical and mental health and wellness.

The journey through this book has unveiled the profound impact of the gut-brain axis. We've discovered that when the mind is in turmoil, the gut echoes this distress. Conversely, an unwell gut creates consequences that disrupt the mind.

The knowledge about this bidirectional communication isn't just a fascinating tidbit of trivia. It's pivotal to our mental health. The gut ecosystem, with its diverse microbial population, is like a musical conductor with an orchestra which together creates an intricate physiological symphony which maintains our physical and mental equilibrium. However, it's a delicate balance, easily tipped by diet, lifestyle, stress, and emotional states.

An imbalanced gut microbiome can lead to systemic inflammation, hormonal disruptions, and even immune system challenges. These may sound like entirely physical ailments, but they're not. They're intertwined with our mental health, creating a cycle in which gut health issues exacerbate mental struggles and vice versa. This interconnectedness underscores a crucial truth: caring for our gut is caring for our mind, and nurturing our mind is nurturing our gut.

This guide has not only provided a wealth of knowledge about the gut-brain connection but also practical strategies to nurture this vital link. The four-part holistic program laid out in these pages – encompassing mindfulness, nutrition, physical activity, and emotional wellbeing – isn't just a plan for gut health or mental wellness; it's a blueprint for a harmonious, balanced life.

Now you've been on this reading journey, you're equipped with tools and insights to cultivate a thriving gut-brain axis as you step forward through life. Whether you start with mindfulness practices, adjust your diet, incorporate physical activity, or enhance your emotional wellbeing, each step is a stride toward holistic health. Remember, there's no one-size-fits-all approach; it's about finding the path to gut health and mental wellness that works for you.

You have the power to make lasting changes, to transform your gut health, your mental state and also your entire being. The knowledge you've gained is your compass, the strategies you have learned are your map. As you embark on this transformative path to health remember, that the journey to wellness is as rewarding as the destination.

So, begin where you are right now, with the choices you make today, and let this be the start of a journey towards a healthier, happier life, where the synergy between gut and mind lays the foundation for a life of wellness and fulfillment.

Free Gut Health Course!

Don't miss out on our exhilarating, FREE course that delves into harnessing gut health for a happier, healthier mind!

Transform Your Life: The Gut-Brain Connection to Mental Wellness

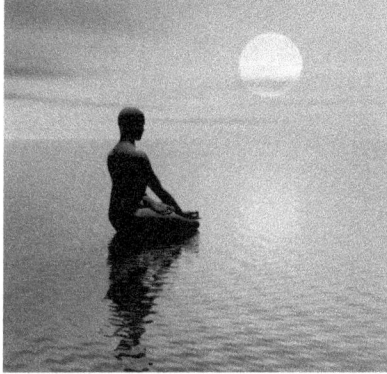

- Unlock the secret to mental wellness with our impactful 10-email course on gut health!
- Learn proven methods to combat stress, anxiety, and depression
- Master mindful eating and stress management
- Build relationships that boost your mental and gut health
- Transform your life with personalized habits for lasting health and happiness

To get your free course, please visit the link or scan the QR code below and let us know the email address to send it to.

pages.healthfitpublishing.com/bonus/fghtmw

Don't miss out!

REFERENCES

"Enteric nervous system: The bridge between the gut microbiota and neurological disorders." by Zi-Han Geng, Yan-Zhu, Quan-Lin Li, Chao Zhao, and Ping-Hong Zhou, National Library of Medicine is licensed under CC BY 4.0

7 easy ways to be mindful in your everyday life. (n.d.). Happify. https://www.happify.com/hd/7-ways-to-be-mindful-in-your-everyday-life/

9 positive mental health habits to try and maintain each week. (n.d.). Believe Perform. https://members.believeperform.com/product/9-positive-mental-health-habits-to-try-and-maintain-each-week/

9 ways gut bacteria and mental health, probiotics and depression are linked. (2020, July 3). Atlas Biomed Blog. https://atlasbiomed.com/blog/9-ways-gut-bacteria-and-mental-health-probiotics-and-depression-are-linked/#vagus-nerve

A quote by L.R. Knost. (n.d.). Goodreads. https://www.goodreads.com/quotes/9180745-taking-care-of-myself-doesn-t-mean-me-first-it-means

Ackerman, C. (2018, April 20). What is positive psychology & why is it important? Positive Psychology. https://positivepsychology.com/what-is-positive-psychology-definition/

Ames, N. J., Barb, J. J., Schuebel, K., Mudra, S., Meeks, B. K., Tuason, R. T. S., Brooks, A. T., Kazmi, N., Yang, S., Ratteree, K., Diazgranados, N., Krumlauf, M., Wallen, G. R., & Goldman, D. (2020). Longitudinal gut microbiome changes in alcohol use disorder are influenced by abstinence and drinking quantity. Gut Microbes, 11(6), 1608–1631. https://doi.org/10.1080/19490976.2020.1758010

Arslan, S. (2020, November 17). What are prebiotics? The complete guide to prebiotics. Omni-Biotic. https://www.omnibioticlife.com/prebiotics-guide/

Bedosky, L. (2022, March 28). Meal planning 101: A complete beginner's guide to meal prep. Everyday Health. https://www.everydayhealth.com/diet-nutrition/meal-planning/

Benefit of yoga. (2018). American Osteopathic Association. https://osteopath-ic.org/what-is-osteopathic-medicine/benefits-of-yoga/

Benjamin Franklin quote. (n.d.). A-Z Quotes. https://www.azquotes.-com/quote/432306

BetterHelp Editorial Team. (2023, October 22). Social comparison: Benefits and risks of comparing yourself to others. BetterHelp. https://www.bet-terhelp.com/advice/general/comparing-yoursel-to-others-downsides-benefits-and-learning-to-love-yourself/

Bhowmik, S. (2023, February 20). How the human gut microbiota is shaped by diet. News Medical Life Sciences. https://www.news-medical.net/news/20230220/How-the-human-gut-microbiota-is-shaped-by-diet.aspx

Bilbray, S. (2014, January 17). Working on your own happiness isn't selfish. Live Happy. https://www.livehappy.com/self/working-on-your-own-happiness-isnt-selfish/

Blanton, K. (2022, March 24). 8 scientific benefits of meal prepping. Everyday Health. https://www.everydayhealth.com/diet-nutrition/scientific-bene-fits-of-meal-prepping/

Bose, P. (2023, March 19). Gut microbiomes and mental health: How do they interact? News Medical Life Sciences. https://www.news-medical.net/news/20230319/Gut-microbiomes-and-mental-health-how-do-they-interact.aspx

Caldwell, A. (2018, June 19). The neuroscience of stress. Brain Facts Organi-zation. https://www.brainfacts.org/thinking-sensing-and-behaving/emo-tions-stress-and-anxiety/2018/the-neuroscience-of-stress-061918

Carver-Carter, R. (2022, May 14). How stress impacts the microbiome and gut health. Atlas Biomed Blog. https://atlasbiomed.com/blog/how-stress-impacts-the-gut-via-the-gut-brain-axis/

Chang, L., & Jing, Y. (2022, April 28). Enteric glial cells in immunological disorders of the gut. Frontiers. https://www.frontiersin.org/arti-cles/10.3389/fncel.2022.895871/full

Chapman, G. (2015, November 13). 5 languages of gratitude. Lifeway Chris-tian Resources. https://www.lifeway.com/en/articles/thanksgiving-languages-of-gratitude

Chassaing, B., Koren, O., Goodrich, J., Poole, A, Srinivasan, S., Ley, R., & Gewirtz, A. (2015, February 25). Dietary emulsifiers impact the mouse gut microbiota promoting colitis and metabolic syndrome. Nature. https://www.nature.com/articles/nature14232

Conlon, M., & Bird, A. (2014). The Impact of Diet and Lifestyle on Gut Microbiota and Human Health. Nutrients, 7(1), 17–44. https://doi.org/10.3390/nu7010017

Couturier, K., & Birmingham, C. (2017, March 27). Yoga for everyone. The New York Times. https://www.nytimes.com/guides/well/beginner-yoga

Creating healthy habits. (2017, December 13). Health Direct. https://www.healthdirect.gov.au/creating-healthy-habits

Definition of selfish. (2018). Merriam-Webster. https://www.merriam-webster.com/dictionary/selfish

Depressive disorder (depression). (2023, March 31). World Health Organization. https://www.who.int/news-room/fact-sheets/detail/depression

Dorsey, A., & 18 WikiHow Co-Authors. (2022, June 9). How to build a healthy relationship. WikiHow. https://www.wikihow.com/Build-a-Healthy-Relationship

Ducrot, P., Méjean, C., Aroumougame, V., Ibanez, G., Allès, B., Kesse-Guyot, E., Hercberg, S., & Péneau, S. (2017). Meal planning is associated with food variety, diet quality and body weight status in a large sample of French adults. International Journal of Behavioral Nutrition and Physical Activity, 14(1). https://doi.org/10.1186/s12966-017-0461-7

Edermaniger, L. (2020, July 3). 9 facts on gut bacteria and mental health, probiotics and depression. Atlas Biomed. https://atlasbiomed.com/blog/9-ways-gut-bacteria-and-mental-health-probiotics-and-depression-are-linked/

Emmons, R. (2019, November 16). Why gratitude is good. Greater Good Magazine. https://greatergood.berkeley.edu/article/item/why_gratitude_is_good

Exercising to relax. (2020, July 7). Harvard Health Publishing, Harvard Medical School. https://www.health.harvard.edu/staying-healthy/exercising-to-relax

Felson, S. (2017, January 26). What are probiotics? Web MD. https://www.webmd.com/digestive-disorders/what-are-probiotics

Firestone, L. (2017, August 17). The unselfish art of prioritizing yourself. Psychology Today. https://www.psychologytoday.com/za/blog/compassion-matters/201708/the-unselfish-art-prioritizing-yourself

Floris, A. (2021, September 1). How does dairy affect gut health? Life Health-care.   https://www.lifehealthcare.co.za/news-and-info-hub/latest-news/how-does-dairy-affect-gut-health/

Food as medicine: Prebiotic foods. (2022, December 21). Children's Hospital of Philadelphia. https://www.chop.edu/health-resources/food-medicine-prebiotic-foods

Foster, J. A., Rinaman, L., & Cryan, J. F. (2017). Stress & the gut-brain axis: Regulation by the microbiome. Neurobiology of Stress, 7, 124–136. https://doi.org/10.1016/j.ynstr.2017.03.001

Freedman, L. (2019, May 29). 10 of our best tips for meal planning for one. The Kitchn. https://www.thekitchn.com/10-of-our-best-tips-for-meal-planning-for-one-242427

Freifeld, L. (2013, March 21). 8 tips for developing positive relationships. Training Magazine. https://trainingmag.com/8-tips-for-developing-positive-relationships/

Fruh, S. M., Mulekar, M. S., Hall, H. R., Adams, J. R., Lemley, T., Evans, B., & Dierking, J. (2013). Meal-Planning Practices with Individuals in Health Disparity Zip Codes. The Journal for Nurse Practitioners : JNP, 9(6), 344–349. https://doi.org/10.1016/j.nurpra.2013.03.016

Fukui, H. (2016). Increased Intestinal Permeability and Decreased Barrier Function: Does It Really Influence the Risk of Inflammation? Inflammatory Intestinal Diseases, 1(3), 135–145. https://doi.org/10.1159/000447252

Geng, Z.-H., Zhu, Y., Li, Q.-L., Zhao, C., & Zhou, P.-H. (2022). Enteric Nervous System: The Bridge Between the Gut Microbiota and Neurological Disorders. Frontiers in Aging Neuroscience, 14. https://doi.org/10.3389/fnagi.2022.810483

Geng, Z.-H., Zhu, Y., Li, Q.-L., Zhao, C., & Zhou, P.-H. (2022, January 17). Enteric nervous system: The bridge between the gut microbiota and neurological disorders. Frontiers. https://www.frontiersin.org/articles/10.3389/fnagi.2022.810483/full

Gill, I. R., & Uno, J. K. (2016). The Impact of Dietary Soy on Gut Microbiome. The FASEB Journal, 30. https://doi.org/10.1096/fasebj.30.1_supplement.1258.2 https://faseb.onlinelibrary.wiley.com/doi/abs/10.1096/fasebj.30.1_supplement.1258.2

Gratitude exercises. (n.d.). Therapist Aid. https://www.therapistaid.com/worksheets/gratitude-exercises

Greatness Authors. (2023, August 5). Is dairy actually bad for your gut health? Here's what both sides have to say. Greatness. https://greatness.com/is-dairy-actually-bad-for-your-gut-health-heres-what-both-sides-have-to-say/

Harpaz, D., Yeo, L., Cecchini, F., Koon, T., Kushmaro, A., Tok, A., Marks, R., & Eltzov, E. (2018). Measuring Artificial Sweeteners Toxicity Using a Bioluminescent Bacterial Panel. Molecules, 23(10), 2454. https://doi.org/10.3390/molecules23102454

Havranek, R. (2022, February 28). 6 ways to exercise improves your gut health. Russell Havranek, MD. https://russellhavranekmd.com/exercise-improves-gut-health/

Heiman, M. L., & Greenway, F. L. (2016). A healthy gastrointestinal microbiome is dependent on dietary diversity. Molecular Metabolism, 5(5), 317–320. https://doi.org/10.1016/j.molmet.2016.02.005

Henry Ford Health Staff. (2021, February 24). How lack of sleep can affect gut health. Henry Ford. https://www.henryford.com/blog/2021/02/sleep-affects-gut-health

Homo sapiens (2021, January 22) The Smithsonian Institution's Human Origins Program. https://humanorigins.si.edu/evidence/human-fossils/species/homo-sapiens

How does social connectedness affect health? (2023, April 3). Centers for Disease Control and Prevention. https://www.cdc.gov/emotional-wellbeing/social-connectedness/affect-health.htm

How stress & anxiety affect your gut. (2022, March 24). Northeast Digestive. https://www.northeastdigestive.com/blog/how-stress-affects-your-stomach/

http://www.behaviorlab.org/Papers/FoodStress.pdf

Kabat-Zinn, J. (2005). Coming To Our Senses. Hyperion Press, NY, NY. https://palousemindfulness.com/docs/bodyscan.pdf

Know your brain: HPA axis. (2014, June 4). Neuroscientifically Challenged. https://neuroscientificallychallenged.com/posts/what-is-the-hpa-axis

Kruis, W., Forstmaier, G., Scheurlen, C., & Stellaard, F. (1991). Effect of diets low and high in refined sugars on gut transit, bile acid metabolism, and bacterial fermentation. Gut, 32(4), 367–371. https://www.ncbi.nlm.nih.gov/pmc/articles/PMC1379072/

Laudisi, F., Stolfi, C., & Monteleone, G. (2019). Impact of Food Additives on Gut Homeostasis. Nutrients, 11(10), 2334.

https://doi.org/10.3390/nu11102334https://www.ncbi.nlm.nih.-gov/pmc/articles/PMC7359750/

Leeming, E. R., Johnson, A. J., Spector, T. D., & Le Roy, C. I. (2019). Effect of Diet on the Gut Microbiota: Rethinking Intervention Duration. Nutrients, 11(12), 2862. https://doi.org/10.3390/nu11122862

Linder, J. (2019, May 9). 5 ways mindfulness practice positively changes your brain. Psychology Today. https://www.psychologytoday.-com/us/blog/mindfulness-insights/201905/5-ways-mindfulness-practice-positively-changes-your-brain

Liu, B.-N., Liu, X.-T., Liang, Z.-H., & Wang, J.-H. (2021). World Journal of Gastroenterology Gut microbiota in obesity Manuscript source: Invited manuscript. World J Gastroenterol, 27(25), 3837–3850. https://doi.org/10.3748/wjg.v27.i25.3837

Mastroianni, B. (2020, May 17). Why Americans are more stressed today than they were in the 1990s. Healthline. https://www.healthline.com/health-news/people-more-stressed-today-than-1990s

Mayo Clinic Staff. (2023, August 10). Stress management. Mayo Clinic. https://www.mayoclinic.org/healthy-lifestyle/stress-management/in-depth/stress-symptoms/art-20050987

McEwen, B. S. (2017). Neurobiological and Systemic Effects of Chronic Stress. Chronic Stress, 1(1), 247054701769232. https://doi.org/10.1177/2470547017692328

McEwen, B. S. (2017). Neurobiological and Systemic Effects of Chronic Stress. Chronic Stress, 1(1), 247054701769232. https://doi.org/10.1177/2470547017692328

Mead, E. (2020, January 14). 8 PERMA model activities & worksheets to apply with clients. Positive Psychology. https://positivepsychology.com/happi-ness-wellbeing-coaching-perma/

Meleen, M. (2022, February 25). Examples of words of appreciation. Your Dictionary. https://www.investopedia.com/terms/a/accountability.asp

Miller, I. (2018). The gut–brain axis: historical reflections. Microbial Ecology in Health and Disease, 29(2), 1542921. https://doi.org/10.1080/16512235.2018.1542921

Mind Tools Content Team. (2022). Active listening. Mind Tools. https://www.mindtools.com/az4wxv7/active-listening

Mind Tools Content Team. (2022). The 7 Cs of communication. Mind Tools. https://www.mindtools.com/a5xap8q/the-7-cs-of-communication

Mind Tools Content Team. (n.d.). Using affirmations. Mind Tools. https://www.mindtools.com/air49f4/using-affirmations

Mindful Staff. (2011, April 20). Why we find it hard to meditate. Palouse Mindfulness. https://palousemindfulness.com/docs/why-we-find-it-hard.pdf

Mindful Staff. (2020, July 8). What is mindfulness? Mindful Communications. https://www.mindful.org/what-is-mindfulness/

Mindfulness-based stress reduction (MBSR). (2019). Palouse Mindfulness. https://palousemindfulness.com/MBSR/week0.html

Mittal, R., Debs, L. H., Patel, A. P., Nguyen, D., Patel, K., O'Connor, G., Grati, M., Mittal, J., Yan, D., Eshraghi, A. A., Deo, S. K., Daunert, S., & Liu, X. Z. (2017). Neurotransmitters: The Critical Modulators Regulating Gut-Brain Axis. Journal of Cellular Physiology, 232(9), 2359–2372. https://doi.org/10.1002/jcp.25518

Monda, V., Villano, I., Messina, A., Valenzano, A., Esposito, T., Moscatelli, F., Viggiano, A., Cibelli, G., Chieffi, S., Monda, M., & Messina, G. (2017). Exercise Modifies the Gut Microbiota with Positive Health Effects. Oxidative Medicine and Cellular Longevity, 2017, 1–8. https://doi.org/10.1155/2017/3831972

Monsivais, P., Aggarwal, A., & Drewnowski, A. (2014, September 18). Time spent on home food preparation and indicators of healthy eating. American Journal of Preventive Medicine. https://www.ajpmonline.org/article/S0749-3797(14)00400-0/fulltext#secsect0055

Muck, P. (2021, September 14). The benefits of yoga: How it boosts your mental health. Houston Methodist. https://www.houstonmethodist.org/blog/articles/2021/sep/the-benefits-of-yoga-how-it-boosts-your-mental-health/

Murphy, E. A., Velazquez, K. T., & Herbert, K. M. (2015). Influence of high-fat diet on gut microbiota. Current Opinion in Clinical Nutrition and Metabolic Care, 18(5), 515–520. https://doi.org/10.1097/mco.0000000000000209

Myers, W. (2014m September 25). 7 great exercises to ease depression. Everyday Health. https://www.everydayhealth.com/depression-pictures/great-exercises-to-fight-depression.aspx

National Heart, Lung, and Blood Institute. (2022, June 15). Sleep Deprivation and Deficiency - How Sleep Affects Your Health | NHLBI, NIH. Www.nhlbi.nih.gov. https://www.nhlbi.nih.gov/health/sleep-deprivation/health-effects

Nieman, D., & Wentz, L. (2019). The compelling link between physical activity and the body's defense system. Journal of Sport and Health Science, 8(3), 201–217. https://doi.org/10.1016/j.jshs.2018.09.009 https://www.sciencedirect.com/science/article/pii/S2095254618301005

Osdoba, K., Mann, T., Redden, J., & Vickers, Z. (2014). Using food to reduce stress: Effects of choosing meal components and preparing a meal. https://doi.org/10.1016/j.foodqual.2014.08.001 Behavioural Lab.

Peden, A. R., Rayens, M. K., & Hall, L. A. (2005). A Community-Based Depression Prevention Intervention with Low-Income Single Mothers. Journal of the American Psychiatric Nurses Association, 11(1), 18–25. https://doi.org/10.1177/1078390305275004. Sage Journals https://journals.sagepub.com/doi/abs/10.1177/1078390305275004

Perry, E. (2022, August 25). 3 types of stress and what you can do to fight them. BetterUp. https://www.betterup.com/blog/types-of-stress

Pinart, M., Dötsch, A., Schlicht, K., Laudes, M., Bouwman, J., Forslund, S. K., Pischon, T., & Nimptsch, K. (2021). Gut Microbiome Composition in Obese and Non-Obese Persons: A Systematic Review and Meta-Analysis. Nutrients, 14(1), 12. https://doi.org/10.3390/nu14010012

Ramdene, H. (2019, May 29). The beginner's guide to meal planning: What to know, how to succeed, and what to skip. The Kitchn. https://www.thekitchn.com/the-beginners-guide-to-meal-planning-what-to-know-how-to-succeed-and-what-to-skip-242413

Robinson, L., & Segal, J. (2020, October). Mindful eating. HelpGuide.org. https://www.helpguide.org/articles/diets/mindful-eating.htm

Rössl, D. (2022, July 19). Is it possible to say no after you said yes already? Path 2 Talent. https://path2talent.com/is-it-possible-to-say-no-after-you-said-yes-already-paulo-coelho/

Sawchuk, C. (2017, June 2). Depression and anxiety: Can I have both? Mayo Clinic. https://www.mayoclinic.org/diseases-conditions/depression/expert-answers/depression-and-anxiety/faq-20057989

Scott, E. (2022, September 19). How to become more mindful in your everyday life. Verywell Mind. https://www.verywellmind.com/mindfulness-exercises-for-everyday-life-3145187

Seven easy ways to include exercise in your daily routine. (2021, September 26). CaroMont Health. https://caromonthealth.org/news/seven-easy-ways-to-include-exercise-in-your-daily-routine/

Sharma, A., Madaan, V., & Petty, F. D. (2006). Exercise for mental health. Primary Care Companion to the Journal of Clinical Psychiatry, 8(2), 106. https://www.ncbi.nlm.nih.gov/pmc/articles/PMC1470658/

Shil, A., & Chichger, H. (2021). Artificial Sweeteners Negatively Regulate Pathogenic Characteristics of Two Model Gut Bacteria, E. coli and E. faecalis. International Journal of Molecular Sciences, 22(10), 5228. https://doi.org/10.3390/ijms22105228

Sidhu, S. R. K., Kok, C. W., Kunasegaran, T., & Ramadas, A. (2023). Effect of Plant-Based Diets on Gut Microbiota: A Systematic Review of Interventional Studies. Nutrients, 15(6), 1510. https://doi.org/10.3390/nu15061510

Sidik, S. (2023, May 25). Chronic stress can inflame the gut – now scientists know why. Nature. https://doi.org/10.1038/d41586-023-01700-y

Smiljanec, K., & Lennon, S. (2019, November 18). Sodium, hypertension, and the gut: does the gut microbiota go salty? American Journal of Physiology. Heart and Circulatory Physiology, 317(6), H1173–H1182. https://doi.org/10.1152/ajpheart.00312.2019 https://journals.physiology.org/doi/full/10.1152/ajpheart.00312.2019

Smith, R. P., Easson, C., Lyle, S. M., Kapoor, R., Donnelly, C. P., Davidson, E. J., Parikh, E., Lopez, J. V., & Tartar, J. L. (2019). Gut microbiome diversity is associated with sleep physiology in humans. PLoS ONE, 14(10). https://doi.org/10.1371/journal.pone.0222394

Splawn, M. (2017, January 19). 10 tips for a happier trip to the grocery store. The Kitchn. https://www.thekitchn.com/10-tips-for-a-happier-trip-to-the-grocery-store-239458

Stress effects on the body. (2023, March 8). American Psychological Association. https://www.apa.org/topics/stress/body

Stress. (2023, February 21). World Health Organization. https://www.who.int/news-room/questions-and-answers/item/stress

Suni, E. (2023, October 25). How to fix your sleep schedule. Sleep Foundation. https://www.sleepfoundation.org/sleep-hygiene/how-to-reset-your-sleep-routine

Sutton, J. (2019, April 9). What is mindfulness? Definition, benefits & psychology. Positive Psychology. https://positivepsychology.com/what-is-mindfulness/#meaning

Sweeney, E. (2023, January 11). Looking to give your gut a little reset?> These 50 probiotic foods are a great place to start! Parade. https://parade.-

com/1043590/ericasweeney/best-probiotic-foods/

Tafet, G. E., & Nemeroff, C. B. (2015). The Links Between Stress and Depression: Psychoneuroendocrinological, Genetic, and Environmental Interactions. The Journal of Neuropsychiatry and Clinical Neurosciences, 28(2), 77–88. https://doi.org/10.1176/appi.neuropsych.15030053 Psychiatry Online. https://neuro.psychiatryonline.org/doi/10.1176/appi.neuropsych.15030053

Tallon, M. (2020, April 13). 10 simple ways to practice mindfulness in our daily life. Monique Tallon. https://moniquetallon.com/10-simple-ways-to-practice-mindfulness-in-our-daily-life/

Thau, L., Gandhi, J., & Sharma, S. (2019, February 15). Physiology, Cortisol. National Library of Medicine; StatPearls Publishing. https://www.ncbi.nlm.nih.gov/books/NBK538239/

The 4 types of stress. (2020, November 10). TELIS Health. https://www.telus.com/en/blog/care-centres/the-4-types-of-stress

The brain-gut connection. (2019). John Hopkins Medicine. https://www.hopkinsmedicine.org/health/wellness-and-prevention/the-brain-gut-connection

The enteric nervous system relays psychological stress to intestinal inflammation. Cell. (n.d.). https://www.cell.com/cell/fulltext/S0092-8674(23)00475-0

The gut and the brain. (2017). Harvard Medical School. https://hms.harvard.edu/news-events/publications-archive/brain/gut-brain

The gut-brain connection. (2023, July 18). Harvard Health Publishing, Harvard Medical School. https://www.health.harvard.edu/diseases-and-conditions/the-gut-brain-connection

The hunger-satiety scale. (n.d.). Berkely University of California. https://uhs.berkeley.edu/sites/default/files/wellness-hungersatietyscale.pdf

The microbiome, stress hormones & gut function. (n.d.). The Institute for Functional Medicine. https://www.ifm.org/news-insights/gut-stress-changes-gut-function/

The surprising link between your microbiome and mental health. (n.d.) Optum. https://www.optum.com/health-articles/article/healthy-mind/surprising-link-between-your-microbiome-and-mental-health/

Thomas, L. (2022, February 7). The effect of diet on mental health. News Medical Health Sciences. https://www.news-medical.net/health/The-Effect-of-Diet-on-Mental-Health.aspx

Tresca, A. (2022, June 9). What is the hypothalamic-petuitary-adrenal (HPA) axis? Verywell Health. https://www.verywellhealth.com/hypothalamic-pituitary-adrenal-hpa-axis-5222557

Volpe, J. (2022, December 19). Prebiotic foods & herbs list PDF (free download). Whole-istic Living. https://wholeisticliving.com/2022/12/19/prebiotic-foods-herbs-list-pdf/

What's the difference between stress and anxiety? (2022, February 14). American Psychological Association. https://www.apa.org/topics/stress/anxiety-difference

Whirledge, S., & Cidlowski, J. A. (2010). Glucocorticoids, stress, and fertility. Minerva Endocrinologica, 35(2), 109–125. National Library of Medicine. https://www.ncbi.nlm.nih.gov/pmc/articles/PMC3547681/

Widener, M. J., Ren, L., Astbury, C. C., Smith, L. G., & Penney, T. L. (2021). An exploration of how meal preparation activities relate to self-rated time pressure, stress, and health in Canada: A time use approach. SSM - Population Health, 15, 100818. https://doi.org/10.1016/j.ssmph.2021.100818

Wikipedia Contributors. (2019, May 12). Psychological stress. Wikipedia, Wikimedia Foundation. https://en.wikipedia.org/wiki/Psychological_stress

Wikipedia Contributors. (2019. Gut-brain axes. Wikipedia; Wikimedia Foundation. https://en.wikipedia.org/wiki/Gut%E2%80%93brain_axis

Wooll, M. (2022, August 2). Find your zen: 15 tips on how to be more patient. BetterUp. https://www.betterup.com/blog/how-to-be-more-patient

Young, C., & Majsiak, B. (n.d.) 5 ways to practice breath-focused meditation. Everyday Health. https://www.everydayhealth.com/alternative-health/living-with/ways-practice-breath-focused-meditation/

ABOUT HEALTHFIT PUBLISHING

HealthFit Publishing is a health and wellness publishing brand. Our mission is to bring sound, actionable knowledge and advice straight from the health and wellness industry to readers from all walks of life. Our focus is on simple lifestyle changes that are easy to make for improving your overall quality of life.

We are made up of a diverse group of dynamic individuals who are passionate about inspiring and motivating others to achieve their health, fitness, and weight loss goals. Our team members are well-respected in their fields and bring expertise and experience in wellness, health, fitness, nutrition, and meticulous research to the table. We are dedicated to making healthy living accessible to anyone who is interested in transforming their life and boosting their happiness by improving their wellbeing.

Our team's diversity is our strong point and the common thread that brings us together is a zest for living life to its fullest and a passion for healthy living. Exercise and good nutrition are just two of our top interests and it's not hard to find inspiration in either.

HealthFit Publishing is the brand behind 'Walking Your Way to Weight Loss', 'Intermittent Fasting for Women', 'Walking Your Way to Weight Loss Plus Intermittent Fasting for Women' 2 in 1 Collection and From Gut Health to Mental Wellness.

ALSO BY HEALTHFIT PUBLISHING

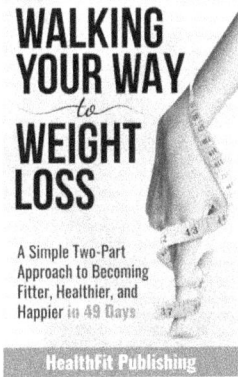

Walking Your Way to Weight Loss: A Simple Two-Part Approach to Becoming Fitter, Healthier, and Happier in 49

Walking Journal & Logbook: A 52-week tracker to capture your daily and weekly progress as you lose weight, achieve fitness and improve health (6" x 9")

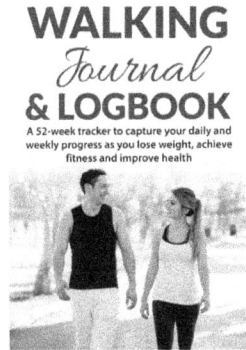

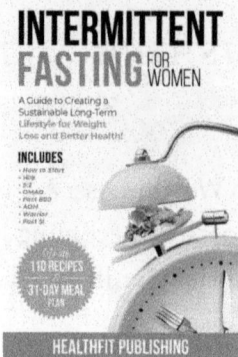

Intermittent Fasting for Women: A Guide to Creating a Sustainable, Long-Term Lifestyle for Weight Loss and Better Health! Includes How to Start, 16:8, 5:2, OMAD, Fast 800, ADM, Warrior and Fast 5!

Walking Your Way to Weight Loss Plus Intermittent Fasting for Women: The Ultimate 2 in 1 Collection for Unlocking the Secrets to Sustainable, Long-Term Weight Loss and a Healthy Lifestyle

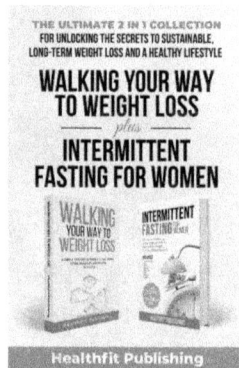

www.ingramcontent.com/pod-product-compliance
Lightning Source LLC
Chambersburg PA
CBHW031547260326
41914CB00002B/313